INFECTION CONTROL PROGRAM GUIDE

Carol Shenold, RN, CIC

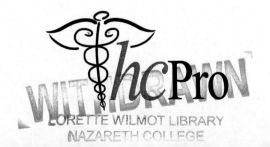

Infection Control Program Guide by Carol Shenold, RN, CIC

Published by HCPro, Inc. Copyright © 2007 HCPro, Inc.

All rights reserved. Printed in the United States of America.　5　4　3　2　1

ISBN 978-1-57839-958-1

HCPro, Inc., provides information resources for the healthcare industry.

HCPro, Inc. is not affiliated in any way with The Joint Commission, which owns the JCAHO and Joint Commission trademarks.

Carol Shenold, RN, CIC, Author
Mary Cresse, Managing Editor
Julia Fairclough, Executive Editor
Bob Croce, Group Publisher
Cindy Robbins, RN, CIC, Reviewer
Jean St. Pierre, Director of Operations
Darren Kelly, Production Coordinator
Leah Tracosas, Copyeditor
Alison Forman, Proofreader
Patrick Campagnone, Cover Designer
Michael Roberto, Layout Artist

Advice given is general. Readers should consult professional counsel for specific legal, ethical, or clinical questions.

Arrangements can be made for quantity discounts. For more information, contact

HCPro, Inc.
P.O. Box 1168
Marblehead, MA 01945
Telephone: 800/650-6787 or 781/639-1872
Fax: 781/639-2982
E-mail: *customerservice@hcpro.com*

Visit HCPro at its World Wide Web sites: *www.hcpro.com* and *www.hcmarketplace.com*

Contents

List of figures

About the author

Carol Shenold, RN, CIC

Carol Shenold, RN, CIC, has worked in healthcare for more than 40 years, many of those spent in acute- and long-term care facilities. She has worked in all hospital departments over the years. During her 12 years as an infection control professional, she specialized in performance improvement, utilization management, and risk management.

In 2003, her employer, Vencor Hospital in Oklahoma City, was recognized for both service and excellence under the Distinguished Hospital Program, a collaborative effort by J.D. Powers and Associates and Health Grades, Inc. The following year she co-hosted HCPro's audioconference, "Infection Control and the 2004 JCAHO Survey Process." In 2005, she served as consulting editor on HCPro's *The CDC's Tuberculosis Guidelines: Key Strategies for Compliance.*

As a freelance author, Shenold has written a column for the OKC *Nursing Times*, served as an editorial advisor for the magazine *Managing Infection Control*, and recently published articles in *Kansas Nurse* and POV by Ethicon.

Shenold writes continuing medical education courses for nurses and speaks to audiences nationwide on the topic of her specialty, bioterrorism.

Introduction

If you're sighing at the prospect of having to read one more handbook on infection control (IC), take heart; I have often felt the same way. Continuous study can be tedious, time-consuming, and frustrating, especially if you are the only person in your department responsible for creating an IC program. It's easy to get overwhelmed. It seems as though every time I turn around, there is a new standard, regulation, or guideline I must memorize.

I've been a nurse in acute care for more than 40 years and an IC practitioner (ICP) for 15. I've worked in hospitals with as few as 30 beds and as many as 300. Been there and done that, from metal bedpans and glass syringes to disposable everything and PDAs with every organism you could want listed in a format you can carry in your pocket. I have never seen the field of IC change so rapidly or so dramatically. So you must believe me when I tell you that you must either create a new infection program now or revise the one that you follow. You, as the ICP, bear the responsibility for ensuring that your staff can speak intelligently about all the current issues in this field. You must believe me when I tell you that, most likely, your policies and plans from as recently as two years ago are outdated.

Here are a few reasons why:

The nurse shortage sets up conditions for an ICP *shortage.* Look around you. Is there anyone in the room beside you? If there is someone beside you in that ICP office, will that person retire soon? Chances are, the answer is yes. The average nurse is in his or her late 40s. If that person is an ICP, likely he or she is preparing to hand the task of creating an IC program to someone else—someone younger, and not yet as well trained.

The role of ICP *has changed.* Years ago, the ICP often served as the "policeman" or "surveillance expert" in the hospital. Now, the ICP is teacher, trainer, student, and compliance officer. He or she must write plans, train staff, and serve on the emergency management committee while maintaining best practices. Moreover, ICPs are under great pressure to formally prove adherence to practice and policy. New tracer methods from The Joint Commission, formerly known as JCAHO, and increased scrutiny from the Occupational Safety and Health Administration (OSHA) are just two reasons IC has moved from protocol to problem.

IC specialists have changed from the person who looked at all the cultures and made certain isolation was reinforced to someone with knowledge of the American Institute of Architects' guidelines for healthcare facilities, soil sampling prior to construction, and the finer points of intermediate sensitivity of a bacteria to specific antibiotics.

Many ICPs are new to their positions. During one recent industry event, a refresher course in the basics of hospital IC, organizers took a poll of the qualifications of ICPs present. There were about 60 attendees; 60% of them had been in their position *for six months or less*. Many said that the IC director role has high turnover. Participants said that they were attending the seminar in part because they needed a refresher in IC principles because they were "thrown into" the position. Many were seeking basic instruction so they could graduate to educating others. Worsening the problem is the common lack of certified ICPs in rural, remote, or small facilities. Therefore, not only are those possessing little or no IC experience hired for the job, those people are expected to accomplish the task as would a veteran, and along with other assigned duties. They may be trying to combine IC with risk management and employee health, each a full-time job in itself.

ICPs *are primed for burn-out.* When people are placed in a position where they must wear nine different hats, including the cap inscribed *Infection Control*, they burn out. I saw a job opening recently for an ICP/Wound Care Nurse. One person, multiple facilities. What a killer position that seems! It wouldn't kill germs; it would kill the nurse trying to oversee any half-decent program in more than one facility.

Your burn-out factor is worsened by the belief among many ICPs that the top brass don't know or don't appreciate what you're doing. Admit it, you agree with me. Maybe this is why administration has no difficulty adding more duties onto or under the IC umbrella—am I correct? Must be, because rarely do additional full-time employees (FTE) enter into that picture. With the added burden of making everything function to meet the Centers for Medicare & Medicaid Services' Core Measures—which greatly contributes to how consumers, regulators, and payers judge the quality of care your facility provides to patients—you are only going to be dancing faster than you are now.

Or have you found that administration wants to place IC in with some other department? In some places, this might comprise a "Quality Department." Perhaps it's an information technology department with support personnel who have IC tasks. Maybe you are working with seasoned IC professionals, but administration is confused because those people may work not only under the title "ICP," but as risk manager, safety officer/director/coordinator, IC nurse/practitioner/officer, facilities management/operations/director, or The Joint Commission survey coordinator.

Despite this, you may also find yourself telling others that that IC concerns are not limited to the IC staff. You must convince others that all departments in a healthcare system are involved in infection prevention, whether by simply being aware of hand-hygiene guidelines or performing as a nurse circulator in surgery. Even The Joint Commission's environment of care program is an integral part of the prevention and control of infections within a healthcare system.

The super staphs and gram-negative bacteria are not only not going away, they're getting worse. Plus, the bird flu is coming. The pernicious spread of *Staphylococcus aureus* within the hospital has overwhelmed us for some time. Even those of us who are skilled in treating communicable diseases—in all settings—can't do much about the infectious diseases that are raging outside hospital walls. Complicating the mix of influences on any IC program are the advent of new and emerging diseases on an almost daily basis, from the Midwest pertussis outbreak in 2006 to the avian flu and the threat of pandemic flu. As if the healthcare-associated infections (HAI) inside the facility were not enough, we must now deal with *community-acquired* infections. Patients now bring into the ED advanced cases of community-acquired methicillin-resistant *Staphylococcus aureus* (CA-MRSA).When CA-MRSA creeps into the hospital, all eyes turn toward us. Where is our plan for dealing with this? Where is our policy? What are we doing to stem the flow of this germ?

Gram-negative bacteria, in particular, is enormously threatening. You simply cannot follow its ever-evolving patterns of antibiotic resistance. Further, many of the new ICPs haven't seen such nasty strains of the bug. Some may know, for example, that the germ is easily transmitted through patient-to-patient contact, but do they know to what extent it is spread to patients by the average healthcare worker (HCW) via hand contact? Do HCWs know what a risk of spread their failure to wash hands creates? My colleagues and I agree that this is a big problem, especially in the intensive care unit (ICU).

HAIs. According to the Centers for Disease Control and Prevention (CDC), about 2 million patients admitted to acute-care hospitals in the United States contract infections unrelated to the conditions that required hospitalization.[1] These infections cause more than 90,000 deaths every year and pump up patient costs by $4.5 billion–$5.7 billion dollars every year.[2] Those figures may change yet again by the time this book goes to print. We'll speak more of HAIs in Chapter 1.

New, intense regulatory attention. The Joint Commission, OSHA, CDC, and others are hyper-aware of the problem and are releasing documents addressing everything from tracer survey preparedness to recommendations for the protection of the spread of communicable diseases. As this book went to press, the CDC announced the release of its final guidelines for isolation precautions and published the new guidelines for handling multidrug resistant organisms.

In 2006, you had to contend with The Joint Commission's unannounced surveys for healthcare facilities in general as well as mid-year self assessments. The Joint Commission also brought the National Patient Safety Goals to prominence as part of the survey process. We've mentioned CMS Core Measures, but did we also mention that they assess surgical infection prevention measures and adherence to such? And that they are publicly reported? Compliance with current CDC hand-hygiene guidelines and self-reporting unexpected infections with poor outcomes as sentinel events are also hot topics. The Joint Commission now requires an infection control construction risk assessment in order to prevent transmission of infections to staff, patients, and visitors due to airborne contaminants like mold. Indoor air quality is another burning issue.

Is there good news in all of this? Yes, of course. As one who is on the crest of major industry change, you have a chance to make a difference. The plan that you create today using this guide could literally save lives.

To do this, you must

- balance all of the features of the IC program, giving all of them the time and attention they need.

- present effective data to assist with change and improvement in the overall IC program. Clear presentation of data can lead to the identification of weak areas in a program or practice and assist in effecting integral changes leading to patient care improvement.

The purpose of this book

The purpose of this handbook is to assist IC professionals in the evaluation and improvement of their own programs, which should include awareness of the conceptual needs of the program under-lain with solid adherence to outside regulatory agencies to keep any program on the right track to continue an effective plan for the prevention and control of infection.

Although this book was inspired by experiences in the healthcare setting, you will find that it has much usefulness in all areas of healthcare. Germs do not discriminate, and neither do we.

You can do it!

I've written over a period of time, I sometimes speak to groups of nurses across the country. When we talk, I realize that IC professionals across the country, in large and small hospitals, have similar problems and are expected to be the experts on everything from head lice to HIV on a 24-hour basis. We will persevere. Hopefully, in some small way, this book will help make your life a little easier. My aim is for this book to include the information you need but not include so much that you can't get through it without hip waders or a snorkel. Hang in there, work with other ICPs, and we'll keep each other from drowning.

It is my hope that this book will provide you with information and ideas to help you develop an excellent IC program and complete a successful Joint Commission survey.

Carol Shenold
Oklahoma City
December 2006

Endnotes

1. CDC, "Monitoring hospital-acquired infections to promote patient safety—United States, 1990–1999," MMWR 49, no. 8 (March 3, 2000):149–153.

2. CDC, "Public health focus: surveillance, prevention, and control of nosocomial infections," MMWR 41, no. 92 (October 23,1992):783–7.

Definitions

The following words and phrases are commonly used in the language of infection control. Compare the list with the acronyms list on page xv.

Annual Assessment – Yearly evaluation of the infection control program and actions taken to prevent and control infections.

Benchmark – A standard or threshold established by data aggregation over a period of time.

C. Difficile – *Clostridium Difficile*, a spore-forming bacteria requiring contact precautions.

CBIC – The Certification Board of Infection Control and Epidemiology, Inc., which provides direction for the certification process for professionals in infection control and applied epidemiology. CBIC is independent and separate from any other infection control-related organization or association.

CIC – Certification in Infection Control, earned by passing an exam administered by the Certification Board of Infection Control and Epidemiology, Inc.

Core Measures – A series of measures designed to affect patient outcomes. They are collected and reported to CMS.

Data Collection – Aggregation of data over a period of time, often to measure patient outcomes.

Data Management – The collection, analysis, display and use of data as a tool for infection control.

Decontamination – The removal of dirt and debris from surfaces, to present a clean surface.

Device Days – The number of days in a period of time, often a month, that a patient is treated with a device such as a ventilator or central line.

Epidemic – A disease outbreak affecting multiple patients or people in a geographical area.

Hand Hygiene – Removing bacteria from hands with soap and water or a waterless product such as alcohol foam.

Healthcare–Associated Infection (HAI) – An infection associated with treatment in a healthcare setting such as a hospital, outpatient facility, long-term care setting, etc.

High Risk – A process or procedure with significant potential for affecting patient safety.

Infection Control Committee – The group of healthcare professionals who form and oversee the management of the infection control program.

Infection Control Practitioner (ICP) – The trained individual who oversees and manages the infection control program.

Infection Control Program – An organized system of services designed to promote the surveillance, prevention, and control of infection.

Infection Prevention and Control – The hospital operations designed to prevent and control healthcare associated infections.

Intervention – Actions taken to prevent or control adverse events such as infection.

Line List – A list of patients, cultures, infections, and risk factors designed to aid in the examination or detection of an outbreak.

Monitor – To observe and record the results of an action in order to assess the effectiveness of the action.

Nosocomial Infection – Hospital acquired, i.e., not present or incubating on admission. Note: Do not use as a synonym for *hospital-associated*.

Outbreak Investigation – The assessment of a cluster of infections to determine the cause and initiate control and prevention measures.

Pandemic – Worldwide disease outbreak—or, a global epidemic.

Rate – A quantitative measure that shows the frequency of an event during a delineated time period.

Resistance – Refers to the ability of a specific bacteria to resist the efforts of an antibiotic.

Risk – The probability of an unfavorable occurrence.

Sentinel Event – An unanticipated and undesirable occurrence that results in, or has the potential to result in, death or serious physical or psychological harm.

Sterilization – The use of a physical or chemical procedure to destroy all microbial life, including highly resistant bacterial endospores.

Surveillance – Continuous monitoring of specific events using an organized and practical approach to identify all occurrences of the event being studied.

Tracers – A session during a Joint Commission survey that evaluates high priority safety and quality of care issues in an organization.

Acronyms

APIC – Association for Professionals in Infection Control and Epidemiology

CABG – Coronary Artery Bypass Graft

CA-MRSA – Community Acquired Methicillin-Resistant *Staphylococcus aureus*

CBIC – Certification Board of Infection Control

CBSI – Central Line-Associated Blood Stream Infection

CMS – The Centers for Medicare & Medicaid Services

DRG – Diagnosis Related Groups

HAI – Healthcare Associated Infections

HIV – Human Immuno Deficiency Virus

ICP – Infection Control Practitioner

MDRO – Multi-drug-Resistant Organisms

MDTB – Multi-drug-Resistant Tuberculosis

MRSA – Methicillin-Resistant *Staphylococcus aureus*

NNIS – National Nosocomial Infection Surveillance

NPSG – National Patient Safety Goal

PFA – Priority Focus Area

PPR – Periodic Performance Review

RFI – Recommendation for Improvement

SCIP – Surgical Care Improvement Program

SIP – Surgical Infection Prevention

TB – Tuberculosis

VAP – Ventilator-Associated Pneumonia

VRE – Vancomycin-Resistant *Enterococcus*

CHAPTER ONE ———————————————————————————————

The infection control program

The rate of healthcare-associated infections (HAI) has reached crisis status in the United States. Every year, 2 million people contract infections unrelated to the condition for which they initially sought treatment; of that number, more than 90,000 people die from these infections every year, according to the Centers for Disease Control and Prevention (CDC). As you create your infection control (IC) program, keep these figures in mind. Also remember this: Although you may not be able to control what occurs outside your hospital, you have much power to control what happens inside your hospital.

In this chapter, you will find the outline of an IC program, within which is a basic IC plan. In subsequent chapters, you will learn how to revise that plan to meet the unique needs of your facility.

See Figure 1.1 for a sample IC plan.

Figure 1.1	SAMPLE INFECTION CONTROL PLAN

INFECTION CONTROL PLAN
Calendar Year 200_

Purpose: The infection control (IC) plan defines the structure and activities for surveillance, prevention, and control of infections among patients, employees, and all others who may come into contact with patients and establishes responsibility for oversight of these activities.

Prioritized Risks are listed in the IC Risk Assessment.

Infection Control Committee Authority Statement: This is a medical staff committee and shall, through its chairperson, the IC nurse (ICN), and all members, have the authority under the medical staff bylaws to institute appropriate control measures when and if an infectious hazard is identified or anticipated that may affect any patient, visitor , or employee. The chairperson and the ICN shall be notified of the potential problem and shall confer with committee members as necessary to institute control measures. In their absence, the director of quality resource management or designee shall assume responsibility for instituting control measures. The IC committee also has the authority for routine identification and analysis of the incidence and cause of all infectious diseases within the hospital and shall develop and implement a plan for the surveillance, prevention, and control of infection hazards.

Goals of the IC program are as follows:
- Keep device-related infections at or below the National Nosocomial Infections Surveillance System (NNIS) rates as per their annual report
- Maintain surgical site infection (SSI) rates at or below the national NNIS rates as per their annual report
- Reach 100% hand-hygiene compliance
- Increase physician compliance with the goals for surgical antibiotic prophylaxis

Strategies to minimize, reduce, or eliminate the prioritized risks are as follows:

Surveillance: The activities related to the IC surveillance plan shall be based on an assessment of the population served in the medical facility, The Joint Commission indicators, high-risk/high-volume indicators, CDC definitions of infections, Medicare's eighth scope of work, surgical infection prevention, and assessed facility needs based on current data collection. County health, state health, and CDC emerging and reemerging disease reports, as well as a reported outbreaks are taken into account when planning surveillance activities. IC activities will add outlying areas to our plan and increase activities at off-site facilities. (See Attachment A. "Infection Control Surveillance Activities")

Orientation and continuing education of personnel: All new employees of this healthcare corporation shall complete an education session presented by the ICN that covers the Bloodborne Pathogen Exposure Control Plan, the Tuberculosis Plan, guidelines for isolation precautions, the CDC's Hand-Hygiene Guidelines and basic IC. Ongoing education will also be provided to employees, physicians, volunteers, patients, and visitors, utilizing a variety of formats and modalities and based on the most current guidelines, regulations, and standards from the

| Figure 1.1 | SAMPLE INFECTION CONTROL PLAN (CONT.) |

The Joint Commission
CDC—Centers for Disease Control and Prevention
OSHA—Occupational Safety and Health Administration
APIC—Association for Professionals in Infection Control and Epidemiology

Isolation/Precautions: All policies related to isolation and precautions are based on the most recent CDC recommendations for standard precautions and airborne, droplet, and contact isolation. *Healthcare Corporation* supports the purchase of necessary supplies and equipment to this end.

Reports to public health officials: Data obtained through surveillance activities shall be appropriately organized and reported to public health officials in a timely manner for their review and action. This includes all "Reportable By Law" diseases to the state department of health, city and county health department(s), and CDC, as appropriate.

IC liaison with employee health: The ICN and the employee health nurse shall act together in the development of policies and procedures related to surveillance, prevention, and control of employee infection, including preemployment health assessments, immunizations, exposures to bloodborne pathogens and other infectious agents, and annual health screening. The employee health department will also collaborate with IC to promote employee vaccination for vaccine-preventable diseases (i.e., influenza). Each will share data and other relevant information and will work with facility employees to create new programs, resolve problems, and promote knowledge of their responsibilities in both departments.

Departmental IC plans: Policies and procedures shall describe activities of prevention and control of infections in all patient care and service areas. All department IC policies and procedures shall be reviewed at least every two years and before as indicated. Reviews will be conducted by department representatives, the ICN, and other experts in related subject matter, using appropriate Joint Commission, OSHA, state/county health department, CDC, and APIC guidelines and regulations. The policies and procedures will be approved by the IC committee. A matrix is presented in the IC manual to show each department's responsibilities.

Engineering controls and waste management: Any engineering controls related to IC, such as negative airflow rooms, surgery suite humidity, building ventilation, waste management, etc., are maintained by Facilities Management, and reports of maintenance, failures, and regulation changes are reported to the IC committee. Policies and procedures for all of these activities are covered by the Facilities Management Department. IC risk assessments will be included for all construction projects deemed appropriate.

Performance improvement study: The Healthcare Performance Improvement Study shall include IC surveillance indicators. These indicators chosen by the IC committee shall be based on appropriate patient and employee populations and treatment modalities of this facility. This performance improvement study is for the express purpose of advancing medical education in the interest of reducing morbidity and mortality among *Healthcare Corporation* patients. Information, interviews, reports, statements, memoranda, or other data relating to the condition and treatment of any person are being used by the Performance

---

| Figure 1.1 | SAMPLE INFECTION CONTROL PLAN (CONT.) |

Improvement Council for the express purpose of advancing medical education in the interest of reducing morbidity and mortality among *Healthcare Corporation* patients and are declared to be privileged communications.

Tuberculosis (TB) control plan: The TB control plan is written to ensure compliance to applicable provisions of the "Guidelines for Preventing Transmission of Mycobacterium Tuberculosis in Health-Care Facilities" published in the *Federal Register* at 58 FR 52810 and shall be based on a TB risk assessment of this facility's patient population, identifying the number of suspected or confirmed infectious TB cases treated in the previous year. The plan establishes guidelines for patient triage, isolation, respiratory protection, education and training of all personnel, TB exposure follow-up, and preemployment and annual employee testing. The plan shall be approved by the IC committee.

Exposure control plan: The exposure control plan shall be written to ensure compliance with applicable provisions of 29 *CFR* 1900.1030, "Occupational Exposure To Blood Borne Pathogens" and shall include guidelines for employee risk assessment by job classification and task, employee education and training, engineering controls, personal protective equipment (PPE), exposure follow-up with related treatment and recordkeeping, and shall be approved by the IC committee.

Disaster plan: IC will help coordinate disaster planning with the safety officer and safety committee for all disasters and potential infectious patient influx conditions.

Construction: All construction in patient areas will receive an IC risk assessment with Facilities Management.

Prevention: Education for staff, patients, and visitors will continue with signs and other methods regarding hand and cough hygiene importance for both staff and visitors as well as isolation and Universal Precautions.

Strategies for prevention will be evaluated in the annual report at the end of each year.

Chairman, Infection Control Committee   Date

In this chapter and throughout this book, we will concentrate on drill-down points. This means, for example, that we will focus on the major points an infection control practitioner (ICP) should know to perform his or her job: The creation and implementation of the IC plan and the related IC department operations and management . The study is up to you. See the "Self-Study" boxes throughout the book.

Now, let's start compiling the basics of an IC plan.

Planning for HAIs: Overview

Vulnerable populations

There are many types of HAIs. Later in this book, you'll find disease-specific recommendations relating to your IC program, but first let's focus on the trends of HAI spread and what victims of HAIs have in common. Frequently, HAI patients are immune-compromised and have multiple comorbidities. Victims are often elderly, although this is not a determining factor—some HAI victims are young, healthy people who became ill while being treated for elective procedures.

Such is the case with MRSA, or methicillin-resistant *Staphylococcus aureus*, victims. As indicated by the CDC, staph infections, including MRSA, occur most frequently among people in hospitals and healthcare facilities (e.g., nursing homes, dialysis centers) who have weakened immune systems. These healthcare-associated staph infections include surgical wound infections, urinary tract infections, bloodstream infections, and pneumonia.[1]

In addition, we must contend with community-acquired methicillin-resistant *Staphylococcus aureus* (CA-MRSA), a strain that can also cause illness in people outside of healthcare facilities. CA-MRSA infections are acquired by people who *have not* recently (within the past year) been hospitalized or undergone a medical procedure (e.g., dialysis, surgery. The CDC has investigated clusters of CA-MRSA skin infections among athletes, military recruits, children, Pacific Islanders, Alaskan Natives, Native Americans, men who have sex with men, and prisoners.[2]

This example of MRSA and CA-MRSA—strains of infection that people can acquire both in and out of healthcare facilities—is just one of many. (See Figure 1.2 detailing the CDC's list of infectious diseases in healthcare settings). And it emphasizes this take-away point: *You must see all patients who enter the doors of your medical facility as potential HAI victims.*

Figure 1.2 | **CDC's LIST OF INFECTIOUS DISEASES IN HEALTHCARE SETTINGS**

According to the CDC, "Healthcare-associated infections (HAIs) are infections that patients acquire during the course of receiving treatment for other conditions or that healthcare workers (HCWs) acquire while performing their duties within a healthcare setting. Specific criteria must be met in order to define an infection as healthcare-associated. In hospitals alone, HAIs account for an estimated 2 million infections and 90,000 deaths annually."

The following are infectious diseases that may be transmitted or acquired in healthcare settings and therefore are possible HAI.

- *Burkholderia cepacia*
- Chickenpox (Varicella)
- *Clostridium Difficile*
- *Clostridium Sordellii*
- Creutzfeldt-Jakob disease (CJD)
- Ebola (viral hemorrhagic fever)
- Gastrointestinal (GI) infections
- Hepatitis A
- Hepatitis B
- Hepatitis C
- HIV/AIDS
- Influenza
- Methicillin-resistant *Staphylococcus aureus* (MRSA)
- Mumps
- Norovirus
- Parvovirus
- Poliovirus
- Pneumonia
- Rubella
- SARS
- *S. pneumoniae* (drug resistant)
- Tuberculosis
- Varicella (Chickenpox)
- Vancomycin-intermediate *staphylococcus aureus* (VISA)
- Vancomycin-resistant *enterococci* (VRE)

 Infection Control Program Guide

Industry and regulatory agencies and HAIs

For more on industry and regulatory agencies, see Figure 1.3.

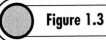

Figure 1.3 — SELF-STUDY: THE BASIS OF YOUR IC RESEARCH

For a successful infection control program, you must stay up to date on the issues. Healthcare industry conferences and events are invaluable resources; however, you may be limited by time and budget and therefore not able to attend them. Set up your own self-study plan that includes focused Web surfing and discussion of IC issues with other professionals both within and outside your facility.

Bookmark these sites in your Web browser and visit them often:

- **CDC**, *www.cdc.gov*
  Start off at the main site, but also go other CDC sites *http://www.cdc.gov/ncidod/dhqp/healthDis.html.* Other CDC sites to visit are the Division of Tuberculosis Elimination (*http://www.cdc.gov/nchstp/ tb/default.htm*) and the page dedicated to the Guidance on Public Reporting of Healthcare-Associated Infections (*www.cdc.gov/ncidod/dhqp/pdf/hicpac/PublicReportingGuide.pdf*).

- ***The Joint Commission***, *www.jointcommission.org*
  If you are not familiar with the *Comprehensive Accreditation Manual for Hospitals*, or *CAMH* (pronounced "Cam"), then seek out your facility's copy and pay particular attention to the standards relating to IC.

  The Joint Commission, as you may note, is involved with other IC organizations—in 2006, it partnered with such organizations as the Association of Professionals in Infection Control and Epidemiology (APIC), the CDC, Society for Healthcare Epidemiology of America (SHEA), the World Health Organization's (WHO) World Alliance for Patient Safety, the Institute for Healthcare Improvement (IHI), and the National Foundation for Infectious Diseases (NFID) to identify best approaches for measuring compliance with hand-hygiene guidelines in healthcare organizations.

- **APIC**, *www.apic.org*
  As stated by the organization: "APIC's mission is to improve health and patient safety by reducing risks of infection and other adverse outcomes. The Association's more than 11,000 members have primary responsibility for infection prevention, control and hospital epidemiology in health care settings around the globe, and include nurses, epidemiologists, physicians, microbiologists, clinical pathologists, laboratory technologists and public health practitioners. APIC advances its mission through education, research, collaboration, practice guidance and credentialing." If you are not a member of APIC, you should join.

Figure 1.3	**SELF-STUDY: THE BASIS OF YOUR IC RESEARCH (CONT.)**

- **SHEA**, *www.shea-online.org*
  Founded in 1980 to advance the application of the science of healthcare epidemiology, SHEA works to maintain the utmost quality of patient care and healthcare worker safety in all healthcare settings. Publications include the quarterly *SHEA News* and *Epidemiology News*.

- **WHO**, *www.who.int/en/*
  The WHO's Web site provides updates on world health conditions, with special sections on disease outbreaks, including disease-specific statistics, such as those on avian flu.

- **HCPro, Inc.**, *www.hcpro.com* and *www.hcmarketplace.com*
  The publishers of this book and leading producers of IC content. On HCPro's Web sites you can order the monthly newsletter *Briefings on Infection Control* and online e-zines *Infection Control Monitor* and *Infection Control Weekly*. You can also find such books as the *Infection Control Manual for Hospitals, Infection Control Compliance Guide, 2nd edition*, and *CDC's Tuberculosis Guidelines: Key Strategies for Compliance*.

The Joint Commission, HAIs, and the Patient Safety Goals

The first standard for hospital accreditation by The Joint Commission requires that hospitals minimize the risk of healthcare-associated infections through the presence of a hospitalwide IC program.

As an ICP, you will come to know well the annual patient safety goals as set out by The Joint Commission—if you don't already. Patient safety goals shed light on problem areas in healthcare that need improvement and lay out proposed solutions to these problems. For example, in 2006, The Joint Commission's goals were set up to help facilities reduce the risk of HAIs and institute IC that would reduce infectious disease acquisition and transmission among hospital staff, patients, and visitors. Pay close attention to the patient safety goals and take a close look at how IC standards are incorporated in your facility, including antibiotic usage, precautions (i.e., safety measures for patients with drug-resistant infections), hand hygiene, cleaning of the facility, and sterilization of instruments and equipment.

Due in part to the increase in HAIs, The Joint Commission initiated the National Patient Safety Goals program. Goal #7 addresses the need for monitoring compliance with hand hygiene in healthcare and recommends the investigation of HAIs that result in death.

     Infection Control Program Guide

In the past, healthcare policy favored keeping news of problems such as HAIs internal. However, increased publicity has made the public aware of the impact of HAIs, and ICPs are expected to be more forthcoming about the topic. Hospitals are encouraged to publicly report infection rates. Visitors to the Web site for the Centers for Medicare & Medicaid Services may access a service called Hospital Compare, set up to help consumers assess how well some hospitals provide care for patients (*www.cms.hhs.gov/ HospitalQualityInits/25_HospitalCompare.asp*).[3] Pay for performance will be based on outcome-related statistics that are publicly reported.

Finding the bones: Elements of a plan

Multiple facets combine to make a comprehensive IC program. The framework for that program includes the following elements:

- A sample written plan that describes
    - the infection risks for the facility
    - strategies to deal with those risks
    - the goals of the program
    - the evaluation plan, i.e., how to evaluate the program
    - surveillance plans for the facility

- Policies and procedures throughout the hospital that affect IC—and how IC might affect policies and procedures throughout the hospital

- Names of individuals who have the authority to take actions to prevent or to control infections

- Reporting systems, which detail how to report infections to
    - appropriate hospital staff
    - state and local public health officials as well as members of the public
    - accrediting bodies, such as The Joint Commission, Occupation Safety and Health Administration, or the Centers for Medicare & Medicaid Services (CMS)
    - organizations receiving patients from the facility

- A sample plan for outbreak investigation

Consideration must be given to many aspects of healthcare that might affect the program. For example, the presence of multiple drug-resistant organisms in hospitals is of great concern, and many of these organisms' occurrence has been the result of antibiotic misuse. Thus, treating infections has become a more complex issue. If hospitals across the country could reduce the use of unnecessary antibiotics, some say, they could save more than $1 billion dollars annually.

Creating a template for handling all IC threats

Diseases that are on the rise, such as the West Nile Virus, severe acute respiratory syndrome (SARS), avian flu, and reemerging diseases such as pertussis and diphtheria, underscore the need for careful consideration of our isolation policies and procedures. The threat of pandemics of influenza or other diseases has prompted us to reevaluate our ability to handle large patient influxes with the systems we now have in place.

HIV and AIDS remain a constant threat in society. In spite of continuing education for adolescents in schools, teen pregnancies remain at an extremely high level, emphasizing the lack of protected sex among young people. Even though the number of AIDS diagnoses is decreasing, populations with limited access to treatment such as the poor and some minorities are seeing an increase in the number of HIV positive people.

Recent events in the United States have further underscored the importance of having a good IC plan in place. The September 11th World Trade Center attacks and subsequent outbreaks of respiratory illnesses believed to be a direct result of the exposure to WTC dust placed more attention on IC and on emergency preparation in the safe operation of a hospital. The added threat of terrorism makes it even more important to educate ICPs not only about how to treat daily outbreaks but also how to treat acts of bioterrorism. Doing so will inform disaster planning and preparation for potential patient influxes, whether from pandemic flu or smallpox. Hurricane Katrina brought to the forefront both the need for hospitals to be able to function independently for long periods of time as well as the need to handle IC issues linked to disaster. For example, rescue workers treating hurricane victims came down with symptoms as varied as norovirus (picked up from infected victims at a Texas refugee camp) and *vibrio vulnificus*, a bacterium present in warm coastal waters that was found to worsen wound infections among rescue workers handling flood situations.

Program structure

Leadership support is crucial for a functional IC program. It helps ensure that the essential financial resources and properly trained frontline and support staff are in place for the IC program to be effective in its goal of infection prevention and control. IC program leaders should aim for the idea of a dynamic, working program. The trained, certified, ICP will be the one who oversees and often enforces infection prevention and control activities as well as data analysis.

ICPs, along with the support of the medical staff director, may delegate specific data collection and infection management tasks to departments such as the pharmacy or nursing units. An IC program must involve multidisciplinary collaboration and implementation. Although not all departments of a hospital may be involved directly in the infection prevention activities, those involved in direct patient care, food handling, environmental services, food service, housekeeping, and laundry services are a few that will be. Anyone who performs direct care or food preparation and services for patients must be involved.

When designing your program, do not stop at regular surveillance issues, such as monitoring the instances of drug-resistant organisms. Include in your plan considerations for such matters as surgical infection prevention measures. Depending upon your hospital's size and status, you may be involved in some of CMS' Core Measure projects, such as the Surgical Care Improvement Project (SCIP), a national quality partnership of organizations committed to improving the safety of surgical care through the reduction of postoperative complications. The ultimate goal of the partnership is to save lives by reducing the incidence of surgical complications by 25% by 2010, according to CMS. SCIP often involves a collaboration between the quality management and IC departments. Core measures data are composed of specific data elements and reflect the clinical performance of the hospital.

As your program evolves, you will discover ways that it needs to be refined to reflect the needs of your facility and community. Completing a sample department matrix, which helps to detail the expectations for various departments, will help you stay focused on the needs of *all* departments.

DEPARTMENTAL IC POLICY MATRIX

	Accounting	Administration	Admitting	Anesthesia	Birth Center	Business Office
Infection Control Policy						
Isolation precautions			X	X	X	
Nonsurgical handwashing	X	X	X	X	X	X
Standard precautions	X	X	X	X	X	X
Employee health						
Work restriction	X	X	X	X	X	X
Health evaluations	X	X	X	X	X	X
TB control	X	X	X	X	X	X
Bloodborne pathogens	X	X	X	X	X	X
Sharps disposal				X	X	
Infectious waste				X	X	
Employee exposure	X	X	X	X	X	X
Department specific						
Sterilization						
Decontamination				X	X	
Disinfection	X	X	X	X	X	X
Food handling					X	
Surgical handwashing					X	

Figure 1.4

DEPARTMENTAL IC POLICY MATRIX (CONT.)

	Cancer Center	Cardiac Rehab	Cardio-pulmonary	CBX	CCU 3	CCU 4	Clinical Equipment
Infection Control Policy							
Isolation precautions	X	X	X			X	
Nonsurgical handwashing	X	X	X	X	X	X	X
Standard precautions	X	X	X	X	X	X	X
Employee health							
Work restriction	X	X	X	X	X	X	X
Health evaluations	X	X	X	X	X	X	X
TB control	X	X	X	X	X	X	X
Bloodborne pathogens	X	X	X	X	X	X	X
Sharps disposal	X	X	X		X	X	
Infectious waste	X	X	X		X	X	
Employee exposure	X	X	X	X	X	X	X
Department specific							
Sterilization	X				X	X	
Decontamination	X	X	X		X	X	X
Disinfection	X	X	X	X	X	X	X
Food handling					X	X	
Surgical handwashing					X	X	

©2007 HCPro, Inc. **13**

The IC committee

Due to the need for many disciplines to be involved in IC, many facilities have chosen to create a multidisciplinary committee to oversee the IC program, take action when outbreaks are identified, sign off on policies and procedures, and be generally involved in drafting the agenda of the meeting and taking the minutes. (Note, however, that not all states require an IC committee.) The IC committee's functions are to assess risks to the facility, evaluate actions that are taken in response to a threat, and recommend actions to take—for example, in situations like an outbreak of C.*difficile*. And after an outbreak, the committee must evaluate the actions taken and recommend further actions as needed.

Multidisciplinary IC Committee

The infection control committee must be multi-disciplinary. Why would it be important to keep the committee diverse? Because a healthcare organization is made up of many disciplines. Each interacts with and supports the other. In the pursuit of infection prevention and control, multiple approaches should be used. In order to make certain all areas of the organization are analyzing their own processes, representatives from all critical areas must be involved, especially those handling direct patient care, whether in cardiopulmonary, surgery, or home health. All areas must be on the same page, collecting and presenting data in the same way.

Departments other than direct care, like nursing and surgery, would be administration for financial and resource support and departments that support direct care—such as environmental services, construction, and the laboratory. It's the cooperation between these departments that maintains a high level of patient safety.

Medical staff involvement is an important element of the IC committee because The Joint Commission will look for it. If you have trouble getting medical staff to attend meetings, sometimes fewer meetings can encourage participation. If you go this route, however, note that some mechanism must be in place for an emergency gathering when needed.

Some departments that should be involved in the IC committee to provide a facility with a well-balanced IC program include

- Nursing
- Laboratory/Microbiology
- Surgery

- Employee Health
- Medical Staff (especially the hospital's epidemiologist and director/program director, infectious diseases)
- Human Resources
- Environment of Care
- Respiratory Therapy
- Pharmacy
- Quality Management
- Other departments as needed or indicated

The goal of this interdisciplinary team is to bring together personnel with expertise in a variety of areas. When this happens, issues can be addressed from multiple angles, and everyone's knowledge enhances the others' abilities. Each member will approach a problem or project from a different aspect—employee training, for example. Let's say you're conducting a training session on multidrug resistant tuberculosis (MDR-TB). The housekeeping department might not need to know details about treatment of the condition, but the laboratorian would certainly need to know more details on the blood assay for M. *tuberculosis* (BAMT). The wise ICP will schedule a meeting with the lab director.

Because a good program is hospitalwide, working together will produce a buy-in that might not be as easily acquired if only one or two departments were involved. Ordinarily, membership on the committee is ongoing, but additional staff members may bring special reports or information as needed. See Figure 1.5 for a sample agenda for an IC committee meeting.

AGENDA

Infection Control Committee
September 2006
Time: 8 a.m.

8:00-8:01: Call to order
8:01-8:10 Review of previous meeting minutes
8:10-8:30 Old business
8:30-9:00 New business:
    1. Surveillance activities:
        1.1 Nosocomial report
        1.2 Resistant organisms
        1.3 Microbiology quarterly report: Not due this month
        1.4 Biological monitoring of sterilizers:
            1.4a Flash percentage
        1.5 Reportable diseases
        1.6 Total renal care, inc. monitors
        1.7 Employee health report
        1.8 Needlesticks report
    2. Isolation monitoring/rounds report: Hand-hygiene compliance
    3. Detailed evaluation of significant infections

9:00-9:30 Other business:
        4.1 Construction: Facilities
        4.2 Home health
        4.3 Procedure review:
            4.3.1 Department procedure review
        4.4 Beta strep infant septicemia
        4.5 West Nile
        4.6 Protect Our Patients Initiative
        4.7 TB assessment
        4.8 Flu letter
Adjournment

The IC committee should be involved in planning, monitoring, evaluating, updating, and educating. It sets general IC policy and provides input into specific IC issues. For example, this committee should routinely review reports from many sources—regulatory agencies, its own facility, medical publications—on hand-hygiene compliance and instances of reportable diseases and outbreaks in making decisions to support its core function on preventing and controlling HAIs. It can accomplish this in a variety of ways, some of which include surveillance of infections, product evaluation, investigation of infection outbreaks and clusters, developing procedures for all departments, patient education, medical waste management, etc.

Successful prevention and control of infection requires careful planning. The IC committee is actively involved in the planning for and implementation of any new procedure that could pose a potential IC risk. For example, if a new construction project is proposed that will involve close proximity of demolition to an immune-compromised population, the committee will review the project and suggest ways to best keep the patients safe from dust and mold.

Note: Depending on the type of facility, the involvement of the IC committee in construction projects varies—although the ICP is in many cases the person who alerts the facility manager to the problem. The ICP might question whether the air exchange in a room is at the proper rate. Such a problem would then be addressed with the facility or plant manager; in other facilities, it might be the safety officer. At one facility I know of, the IC director works with the engineering department. Together they review the IC construction assessment (ICRA) for each project to provide for the safety of patients and staff. See Chapter 2 for an example of an ICRA.

The IC committee also may provide input into the selection of chemicals used to manage the environment, such as detergents and disinfectants. For example, many housekeeping departments or a professional cleaning service may use certain products most often, and those products will have to be listed and reviewed by the committee for rejection or approval of its use.

The committee also monitors infectious processes within the healthcare facility. It tracks HAIs and incidents that have the potential to cause infections. It reviews its facility's surveillance program and recommends changes as needed. It also reviews the facility's year-end report and helps decide whether the program's overall focus needs to change due to new threats or outbreaks of infection in new areas.

While monitoring specific incidents, the IC committee keeps an eye toward the bigger picture as it continually strives to improve processes within the facility. This is demonstrated by the regular review of IC procedures for all departments, as well as the periodic evaluation of practices and offering input regarding products and protocols.

One of the biggest challenges that all IC committees face is keeping current. The constant advancement of medical technology introduces changes at all levels within the healthcare facility, new bacterial strains complicate and challenge older IC practices, and new research often requires reexamination of established procedures. The IC committee's purpose is to provide guidance and leadership through these changes. All members of the team must strive to keep abreast of changes within their area of expertise.

Finally, as an integral part of its leadership, the committee must take an active role in staff education. That role may be a hands-on approach or it may be an advisory role in partnership with the facility's education department. However it functions, the committee must set direction for both staff education and validation of that education.

The staff education process should at least address two specific areas: general IC education and continual updating. The first educational need, general IC education, is usually accomplished through an annual education program designed for all employees. The annual program should provide the groundwork for general IC protocols, which create a safe environment for both patients and employees. Information covered by this program might include standard bloodborne pathogen education, rules laying out proper use of personal protective equipment (PPE), etc.

The second educational need that the IC committee addresses is communicating updated information. In the constantly changing healthcare arena, the committee must find a way to make sure the entire hospital staff is aware of changes in information. This is usually done through inservices, newsletters, or published committee communications, such as meeting minutes. Whatever the method, the goal is to create a smooth flow of information to all employees.

Both of the IC committee's educational roles should focus on creating awareness of IC and developing the skills necessary to function effectively on the job among staff. Daily (if possible) surveillance rounds on units or floors to observe the use of PPE or signage that instructs others in precautions should be in place. Ideally, staff training should be one-on-one so the trainer can spot and stop wrong behavior.

Everyone knows that IC is the responsibility of all healthcare workers: Patients and employees are only safe from infectious processes when everyone follows good IC techniques. The purpose of the IC committee is not to reduce the individual responsibility that each healthcare provider has but to provide leadership for all employees throughout the facility. Through policies, procedures, and evaluation processes, the committee acts as a central clearinghouse for all IC information, channeling that information in a manner that will create the safest healthcare environment.

The committee also helps to standardize IC procedures throughout the facility so the same level of care is provided in all departments. The fewer procedures in place that only apply to specific departments, the better. For example, the IC committee should take steps to ensure that the standard for cleaning laryngoscopes is the same in the operating room as it is in the cardiopulmonary department, the cath lab, minor procedures unit, and the emergency department.

In addition to providing or recommending formal educational opportunities, the IC committee communicates with employees through the use of procedures. The committee must maintain written IC procedures, which should be available to all employees. Many companies have their IC manual on the hospital's intranet, eliminating the need for constantly updating multiple paper manuals.

In addition to channeling information through itself, the committee acts as a facilitator between other departments, often coordinating communication between departments to smooth the sharing of information and procedures.

The purpose of the IC committee is simple: to prevent and control infection. Achieving that goal requires the skills and input of the many healthcare disciplines serving on the committee and the cooperation of all employees. The committee is designed to provide clear direction to help everyone create and maintain a safe environment.

Endnotes

1, 2. Centers for Disease Control and Prevention. Site, "Community Associated MRS Information for Clinicians." Accessed December 6, 2006. *www.cdc.gov/ncidod/dhqp/ar_mrsa_ca_clinicians.html*.

3. According to a statement from the U.S. Department of Health & Human Services, "Hospital Compare is a consumer-oriented website that provides information on how well hospitals provide recommended care to their patients. On this site, the consumer can see the recommended care that an adult should get if being treated for a heart attack, heart failure, or pneumonia or having surgery. The performance rates for this website reflect care provided to all U.S. adults.

"This website was created through the efforts of the Centers for Medicare & Medicaid Services (CMS), along with the Hospital Quality Alliance (HQA). The Hospital Quality Alliance (HQA): Improving Care Through Information was created in December 2002. The HQA is a public-private collaboration established to promote reporting on hospital quality of care. The HQA consists of organizations that represent consumers, hospitals, doctors, employers, accrediting organizations, and federal agencies. The HQA effort is intended to make it easier for the consumer to make informed healthcare decisions, and to support efforts to improve quality in U.S. hospitals. The major vehicle for achieving this goal is the Hospital Compare Web site." (Site accessed December 14, 2006.)

Identifying facility risks

Risks change over time—sometimes quite rapidly. Assessment of your hospital's infection risks should be ongoing, with formal analysis annually, at the least. In addition, if your facility adds a new service or begins performing invasive procedures in a new area, you need to address those risks. For example, if your facility adds bariatric surgery to its ambulatory services department, what new infection surveillance might be needed that wasn't necessary in the past? Or if a new corrections facility is built nearby, would your population mix of the patients change or would this add new disease potentials to your community?

Risks for infection vary in every facility. The best way to tailor your infection control (IC) program is by assessing the risks present in the facility's brick-and-mortar buildings. Many elements may be part of your program evaluation depending upon a variety of aspects. Some elements that will affect a healthcare facility include

- geographic location
- community environment
- services provided
- population served

Risks associated with facility location

What kind of risk does your hospital run that would be related to location? Are you near the ocean or land locked? Is your emergency department more likely to see patients with frost bite, snake bites, or jelly fish stings?

If you live in Oklahoma, for example, you're familiar with tornadoes. You know that hospital care during a tornado is difficult to maintain. Initially, this is not an infection control (IC) problem;

©2007 HCPro, Inc.

at the onset and in the days after you're more concerned with, for example, interruption of electrical service, emergency response, injuries common to the onset of tornadoes, and the other health problems that attend destruction of an area. In the aftermath, you will begin to see more IC-related problems. Infection could be a factor if the destruction means a large influx of patients, increased mortality with no way to efficiently take care of bodies—a surge in the emergency department that presents ideal conditions for spread of disease, be it norovirus, the seasonal flu, or our old friend CA-MRSA, community acquired methicillin-resistant *Staphylococcus aureus*.

Even before the onset of Hurricane Katrina, the residents of the U.S. Gulf Coast lived with flooding left by hurricanes. Even without disruptions in utilities, travel, and communication, standing water increases the risk of mold formation and waterborne diseases. This was true after Katrina. In fact, more than a year after the onset of the storm, many Gulf Coast residents were working on houses that had to be torn down or rebuilt in part because of the damage due to mold. Mold can be especially pernicious because it remains in buildings long after the water has gone.

In the desert Southwest, diseases such as the Hanta virus and the plague are endemic and can be seen in the rodent population. All of these scenarios have the potential for putting a facility at risk, but all hospitals will not have the same risks.

Figure 2.1 | **INVOLVING THE ICP IN PROJECT PLANNING**

Architects, contractors, and facility managers don't have a long history of working with infection control professionals (ICP) to protect patients—not from a lack of desire, but rather from a lack of awareness of the risk. Now that the AIA and The Joint Commission have included the need for patient safety and completion of the infection construction assessment (ICRA) in their guidelines, both administration and facilities management have become more accepting of involving ICPs in construction planning from the beginning of the project.

All facilities need to prevent mold-related outbreaks from occurring whenever possible. That doesn't mean incidents won't occur in spite of precautions. There's no guarantee that structural changes won't lead to moisture entering a building and posing a potential for mold growth. It does mean, however, to avoid activities that can cause mold to grow or allow mold spores to disperse into the air. When those activities cannot be avoided, take appropriate measures to contain any dust produced.

Prevention is the key to the ICRA. The ICRA identifies the patient populations housed in the areas under construction. Under the ICRA, evaluate the type of project to determine whether it will simply involve using new materials to construct a wall or whether it calls for demolition of walls, transportation of debris, etc. Once you have identified the patient population and type of construction, discuss measures needed to protect that population.

| Figure 2.1 | INVOLVING THE **ICP** IN **PROJECT PLANNING** (CONT.) |

Project planning is done during a sit-down meeting with all interested parties, including the infection control nurse, architect, safety officer, facilities manager, and heads of affected departments. Some facilities include the vice president in charge of finance. In this meeting, discussion begins using floor plans to review the exact nature of the job. Address many aspects of the project at this or at future meetings. Document the meetings in the form of minutes and on the risk assessment form itself. Keep copies of the documentation in both the infection control office and facilities management office.

The team developing the ICRA provides ongoing planning during the entire project, especially throughout the demolition, construction, cleanup, and preparation to resume services. Initially focus on isolation of the area in terms of minor or major risks, based on the level of needed barriers.

The risk assessment determines the types of barriers needed and accounts for the degree of activity, level of dust generated, and proximity to patients with varying levels of risk for infection. Internal renovations can require as much consideration of infection control as external ones. Patient areas that cannot be closed off, such as operating rooms, require special planning. If possible, conduct external excavations during off hours so air handlers can be shut down, thus reducing risks to patients.

Some measures can be taken to control mold-contaminated dust and debris. Include them in the ICRA. The complexity of these measures is based on the patient population in the construction area or in close proximity, including the following:

- Removing medical waste containers before the start of the project
- Installing barriers to prevent dust from entering
- Limiting removal of ceiling tiles to one at a time when possible
- Sealing air-handling systems between areas
- Creating negative air pressure
- Controlling foot traffic
- Removing waste in covered carts
- Sealing windows
- Monitoring daily for compliance

from Healthcare Mold Management, by Carol Shenold and Mark Hodgson (HCPro, 2004)
Available through hcmarketplace.com

Community environment

It can be difficult to separate geographic location and the less tangible "community," or community environment. The specific ethnicity of a community, social patterns, and other ingredients in the cultural mix combine with factors that make minor risks in, say, a rural community very real risks in an urban community. For example, in a rural setting, a facility could run the risk of cutaneous anthrax due to animal skinning. Anthrax being a risk might not be due to the threat of bioterrorism as much as the lifestyle and livelihood of the local population. Within an urban area, there might be a higher risk of sexually transmitted diseases like HIV and AIDS and hepatitis B; hepatitis C and tuberculosis can be found in the general urban population as well as the high-risk populations found commonly within cities, notably the homeless, chemically dependent, those released from prison, and the mentally ill.

Services provided

Not all hospitals are full-service providers. A specialty hospital that is long-term acute-care facility may not deal with the patient population seen in a short-term acute-care facility that has obstetric and surgical services. However, a facility that has long-term ventilator patients, often seen in long-term acute services, might have a greater risk of ventilator associated pneumonias (VAP). An acute-care facility has a much greater potential for a large number of flu patients to be admitted during flu season. These dynamics influence choices in IC surveillance.

Never discount the threat posed by stand-alone entities in an organization. The presence of an outpatient wound care center, behavioral health treatment facility, or rehabilitation clinic can add infections that must be addressed in the overall risk assessment due to the presence of high-risk populations.

Populations

When assessing risks that your population might pose, consider both patients in your hospital and those who are likely to be admitted to your hospital populations. For example, if your hospital has a neonatal intensive care, you have an internal population that could be placed at risk by something as simple as artificial fingernails or beta strep infection in the mother. Also consider what neighborhoods surround you. Do you have a large number of nursing homes in the same area? You may run a higher risk of methicillin-resistant *Staphylococcus aureus* (MRSA) than a hospital in another area due to the demographics of your admissions.

Ethnic mix can also affect the types of infections you see simply because of an occupation favored by a particular group or a susceptibility to diabetes that increases the risk of postoperative infection.

Cultural differences may also affect the likelihood of a particular population's participation in preventive healthcare. For example, some groups don't avail themselves of healthcare systems until there are no choices left.

The economic mix of a population may also affect the infection risks in a particular area. For example, in uninsured populations, a risk exists for patients to ignore health problems when they could be easily treated. That, in turn, can lead to longer lengths of stay with increased risk of healthcare-acquired infections.

Visitors

Most healthcare organizations don't try to follow infections in visitors as such. But always be aware of the potential risk of visitors bringing infections into or carrying infections away from a hospital. For instance, The Joint Commission has stated that several organizations dealing directly with the SARS epidemic in Canada noted that they should have moved more quickly to limit visitors and thus reduce the risk of spreading infection.

Risk assessments: Forms and types

Even a simple form of risk assessment can lend focus to an IC plan and allow an organization to funnel its resources into the areas of greatest need. Creating a risk assessment is your way of quantifying the probability of a harmful effect to individuals or populations from certain activities. Risk assessments can take all forms—and not all are IC-related. However, some involve IC concerns: For example, a security risk assessment might address IC in the context of surge capacity—that is, the hospital's vulnerability in allowing infectious populations from outside to enter the hospital. Other risk assessment involving IC include

- **condition-specific**, such as in an IC construction risk assessment (ICRA) (see Figure 2.3, "Infection control risk analysis," and Figure 2.4, "Infection control risk assessment/matrix of precautions for construction and renovation," at the end of this chapter)

- **disease-specific**, such as in a tuberculosis (TB) risk assessment (see Figure 2.5 at the end of this chapter).

The risk assessment should be presented to the IC committee (ICC). That way, as the annual IC program analysis is completed, the results of all risk assessments can be incorporated into the program, and the assessments will be funneled up to the medical staff committees and the executive board.

Because risk assessments for IC are performed annually, the process could be structured in a couple of ways. You could cluster assessments to be due at the same time of year or space them out to be performed, for example, on a quarterly basis. Note that the TB risk assessment is an assessment you need to do routinely. It also has an annual requirement. ICRAs can be done on a schedule or as needed, depending upon the status of your hospital's construction. But first let's address the TB risk assessment.

TB risk assessment

The idea behind the TB risk assessment is to analyze your hospital's TB control program and its ability to control the spread of TB among patients, visitors, and employees.

The Occupational Safety and Health Administration (OSHA) revised its TB guidelines at the end of 2005. Those guidelines spell out what OSHA expects to see in the annual assessment. The administration also changed some of the requirements for routine TB testing for hospitals that are assessed at a low risk for contact with patients who have active TB.

If your organization's risk appears to be low, keep in mind that it only takes one TB case to put your facility at risk. In September 2006, an Oklahoma hospital discovered that one of its employees had active TB. The employee had worked on several units and exposed multiple patients, visitors, and employees. Letters were sent to patients, the incident leaked to the media, and everyone who went near the facility in the fall wanted to be tested. In a similar case in 2005 in Boston, a surgical resident who rotated through four Massachusetts hospitals while she had a contagious form of the disease for six months exposed thousands to the germ. These were only two cases, and cases that were not hidden from the public. Let this serve as a warning: Even if you find your facility's TB risk to be low, carefully consider your options before deciding not to continue annual employee testing. If you regularly test employees who have direct patient contact, you at least have baseline testing in place for one group.

Included under the risk assessment umbrella is also product assessment. For the general IC program, assessment might include analysis of anything from new safety needles, antibiotic-impregnated catheters, and hand disinfectants to environmental cleaning products. Any environmental cleaners should be approved through the ICC.

Performing the risk assessment

OSHA's guidelines want to see TB risk assessments performed for all settings in your organization, even the nontraditional ones, such as freestanding outpatient surgery centers, HIV/AIDS clinics, or home health. Some of the factors you need to take into consideration in your assessment are

- TB skin test conversion rates for each setting
- environmental controls in place in each setting
- the numbers of active TB cases encountered annually in each setting
- the length of time between when a patient with suspected TB is admitted and when that patient is placed in airborne isolation
- the time between ordering sputum cultures, collecting them, sending them to the laboratory, receiving results, and calling critical results to a physician
- the number of negative-pressure isolation rooms in the facility
- air exchanges in negative-pressure isolation rooms
- preventive maintenance on the negative-pressure systems and their monitoring

Also review OSHA's TB guidelines, as well as the sample assessment on p. 34. For more information on TB guidelines, pick up HCPro's book *Understanding OSHA's Tuberculosis Guidelines*.

Keep in mind that any hospital or setting with an assessment risk level above no or low risk must continue to perform TB skin tests on at least an annual basis or more often, as well as fit test TB masks annually.

Linking facility safety to immunity risks

Also extremely important for your facility's overall control of risks is the strict performance of the Infection Construction Risk Assessment, often called ICRA. Performing this assessment allows you to be certain that you are preventing and controlling any potential for your patients to be exposed to mold or harmful air particles produced during construction or demolition occurring in or on your property. Even if the construction does not involve a major project or demolition, the simple act of removing ceiling tiles and pulling cable can dislodge dust, mold, or debris. With the ICRA, you, the engineering staff, and the construction boss have to agree upon the measures you plan to use to protect your patients.

When to perform an ICRA

There is no requirement for use of a particular ICRA tool or form. The Joint Commission's Environment of Care (EC) chapter says, in the element of performance EC.8.30, that a proactive risk assessment is to be performed to minimize risk to the patient any time a space is renovated, altered, or newly created. There are several excellent sources of information and tools available. These include matrices that classify construction projects by types and activities; descriptions of required infection control precautions by class (both during construction and upon completion of your project); and hard-copy forms that ask for the signatures of contractors and subcontractors.

Each facility has to assess the need for an infection control risk assessment by the potential for close proximity of the project to a high-risk patient population and the potential for release of dust/debris/mold into the air. Even the removal of ceiling tiles for pulling electrical cables could pose a risk. Any new project should be evaluated as to the need for patient protection.

The ICRA must be comprehensive in scope and deal with patient relocation, barriers limiting airborne contaminants, and air-handling or water systems that regulate airborne and waterborne pathogens. These steps take on added significance because the AIA guidelines now require the "phasing" of construction and renovation projects to minimize patient and staff exposure to potential contamination. Phasing allows you to keep exposure limited to small areas and time frames by completing a portion of a project before beginning the next phase.

Each ICRA must be specific to one project and address a wide range of issues. Work closely with your facilities planner, architect, and contractor to make certain everyone involved understands his or her role in infection control. Elements the ICRA considers, especially for populations susceptible to airborne contaminants like mold, are:

- Patient population
- Facility programs
- Disruption of essential services
- Patient placement or relocation
- Effective barriers to protect susceptible patients from Aspergillus sp or other mold-related diseases

Criteria used for categorizing patients should include patient susceptibility to infection as well as identifying invasive procedures performed in the construction area. Classifying projects helps you determine how much dust will be created. Patient groups are matched with project categories to select the level of required precautions.

During the design phase of a project, for example, your architect and facility manager should plan for the placement of barriers to isolate specific areas during construction. Your contractor, in turn, will be responsible for actually erecting the barriers. You can use a wide range of materials, including fire-rated plastic and temporary walls, with doors that seal.

Architects, contractors, and facility managers may not have much experience working with infection control professionals (ICP) to create environments that protect patients—not from a lack of desire, but a lack of awareness of the risk. Now that the AIA and The Joint Commission have included the need for patient safety and completion of the ICRA in their guidelines, those who work in both administration and facilities management are more accepting of the necessity involving the ICP in construction planning.

As you consider the patient populations at risk, you will assess the immune status of the groups closest to, and thus most likely to be affected by, the construction. The ICRA will allow you to tailor your precautions to the affected population. Measures might include some or all of the following:

- Covering trash during transport
- Alternating hours for construction activity
- Using walk-off mats
- Setting up barriers, such as visquene or temporary walls
- Improved egress design (i.e., directing traffic flow in the area)
- Use of high-efficiency particulate air filter (HEPA) vacuum for clean-up
- Temporary transfer of patients to another area
- Use of negative-pressure construction areas
- Shoe covers for construction workers

While you perform ICRAs with the facilities department, produce IC construction permits and have them available and easily accessible for regulatory agencies. See Figure 2.2 for a sample IC construction risk assessment and permit.

Make full use of the statistics available through your city/county health department, your state health department, and other regulatory agencies such as OSHA, The Joint Commission, Centers for Disease Control and Prevention, and the World Health Organization. This way, you will have those numbers that lend credibility to the decisions you make when choosing your surveillance activities and employee health procedures.

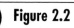

Figure 2.2

INFECTION CONTROL CONSTRUCTION PERMIT

Location of Construction: 3 South
Project Coordinator:
Contractor Performing Work
Supervisor:

Permit No:20052
Project Start Date: 11-01-2005
Estimated Duration:
Permit Expiration Date:
Telephone:

Yes	No	Construction Activity	Yes	No	Infection Control Risk Group
		TYPE A: Inspection, non-invasive activity			GROUP 1: Low Risk
X		TYPE B: Small scale, short duration, moderate to high levels		X	GROUP 2: Medium Risk
		TYPE C: Activity generates moderate to high levels of dust, requires greater 1 work shift for completion			GROUP 3: Medium/High Risk
		TYPE D: Major duration and construction activities Requiring consecutive work shifts			GROUP 4: Highest Risk

Class I	1. Execute work by methods to minimize raising dust from construction operations. 2. Immediately replace any ceiling tile displaced for visual inspection.	3. Minor Demolition for Remodeling
Class II	1. Provides active means to prevent airborne dust from dispersing into atmosphere. 2. Water mist work surfaces to control dust while cutting. 3. Seal unused doors with duct tape. 4. Block off and seal air vents. 5. Wipe surfaces with disinfectant.	6. Contain construction waste before transport in tightly covered containers. 7. Wet mop and/or vacuum with HEPA filtered vacuum before leaving work area. 8. Place dust mat at entrance and exit of work area. 9. Remove or isolate HVAC system in areas where work is being performed.

Figure 2.2	**INFECTION CONTROL CONSTRUCTION PERMIT** (CONT.)

Class III	1. Obtain infection control permit before construction begins. 2. Isolate HVAC system in area where work is being done to prevent contamination of the duct system. 3. Complete all critical barriers or implement control cube method before construction begins. 4. Maintain negative air pressure within work site utilizing HEPA equipped air filtration units. 5. Do not remove barriers from work area until complete project is thoroughly cleaned by Env. Services Dept. tightly covered containers. 6. Vacuum work with HEPA filtered vacuums. 7. Wet mop with disinfectant. 8. Remove barrier materials carefully to minimize spreading of dirt and debris associated with construction. 9. Contain construction waste before transport in tightly covered containers. 10. Cover transport receptacles or carts. Tape covering. 11. Remove or isolate HVAC system in areas where work is being performed.
Class IV	1. Obtain infection control permit before construction begins. 2. Isolate HVAC system in area where work is being done to prevent contamination of duct system. 3. Complete all critical barriers or implement control cube method before construction begins. 4. Maintain negative air pressure within work site utilizing HEPA equipped air filtration units. 5. Seal holes, pipes, conduits, and punctures appropriately. 6. Construct anteroom and require all personnel to pass through this room so they can be vacuumed using a HEPA vacuum cleaner before leaving work site or they can wear cloth or paper coveralls that are removed each time they leave the work site. 7. All personnel entering work site are required to wear shoe covers. 8. Do not remove barriers from work area until completed project is thoroughly cleaned by the Environmental Service Dept. 9. Vacuum work area with HEPA filtered vacuums. 10. Wet mop with disinfectant. 11. Remove barrier materials carefully to minimize spreading of dirt and debris associated with construction. 12. Contain construction waste before transport in tightly covered containers. 13. Cover transport receptacles or carts. Tape covering. 14. Remove or isolate HVAC system in areas where work is being done.

Additional Requirements:

_____ Exceptions/Additions to this permit are noted by attached memoranda

_____ _____
Date   Initials

Permit Request By:

Permit Authorized By:

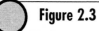 **Figure 2.3**

SAMPLE INFECTION CONTROL RISK ANALYSIS

Infection Control Risk Analysis
2006

The potential risks and threats to _____ Hospital patients, licensed independent practitioners, staff, volunteers, students/trainees, visitors, and families from an IC perspective.

Information from facility, state, and national resources used to make decisions, i.e. state statistics for STD, CDC statistics, and local surveillance reports.

Threat probability: 1–5, with 1 being least likely and 5 being imminent danger.

Type of Infection Event	Probability of Incident Occurring	Internal Resources Available	External Resources Available
Bioterrorism	2	Disaster plan	Communitywide exercises and drills
Epidemic, external	2	Multiple disaster plans with overall plan developing	Communitywide awareness
Epidemic, internal	2	Continual monitoring and surveillance for important diseases and syndromes as identified	Public health surveillance
Influenza	4	Standard plan for droplet precautions continues in effect along with hand- and cough-hygiene reminders. Continuing patient and employee vaccination campaigns.	State health department surveillance
Influenza pandemic	3	Would trigger the disaster plan if it hit this state in disaster numbers	State health department and CDC resources
Bloodborne pathogens	4	Bloodborne pathogens plan and standard precautions	
C. difficile	4	Standard and contact precautions, hand hygiene	
SARS	2	SARS plan	State health department and CDC resources

 Infection Control Program Guide

Figure 2.3	SAMPLE INFECTION CONTROL RISK ANALYSIS (CONT.)

Type of Infection Event	Probability of Incident Occurring	Internal Resources Available	External Resources Available
TB	3	TB plan with all precautions in place.	State Health department and CDC resources
IC sentinel event	3	Risk management and root-cause analysis	
Surgical site infections	3	SIP interventions	National SIP project
CBSI	3	Surveillance	NNIS data
VAP	3	Surveillance	NNIS data
FUTI	3	Surveillance	NNIS data
UAC	3	Surveillance	NNIS data
Beta strep septicemia newborns	2	Surveillance	
MRSA	4	Standard Precautions and Contact Precautions, hand hygiene	State health department and CDC resources, internal surveillance
VRE	4	Standard contact precautions, hand hygiene	State health department and CDC resources, internal surveillance
Employee outbreaks	3	Employee health procedures	

⬤ **Figure 2.4** | **INFECTION CONTROL RISK ASSESSMENT**
MATRIX OF PRECAUTIONS FOR CONSTRUCTION & RENOVATION

Step 1:
Using the following table, *identify* the **Type of Construction Project Activity (Type A-D).**

Type A	**Inspection and non-invasive activities.** Includes, but is not limited to: • removal of ceiling tiles for visual inspection limited to 1 tile per 50 square feet • painting (but not sanding) • wallcovering, electrical trim work, minor plumbing, and activities that do not generate dust or require cutting of walls or access to ceilings other than for visual inspection
Type B	**Small scale, short duration activities which create minimal dust** Includes, but is not limited to: • installation of telephone and computer cabling • access to chase spaces • cutting of walls or ceiling where dust migration can be controlled
Type C	**Work that generates a moderate to high level of dust or requires demolition or removal of any fixed building components or assemblies** Includes, but is not limited to: • sanding of walls for painting or wall covering • removal of floorcoverings, ceiling tiles, and casework • new wall construction • minor duct work or electrical work above ceilings • major cabling activities • any activity cannot be completed within a single workshift
Type D	**Major demolition and construction projects** Includes, but is not limited to activities that: • require consecutive work shifts • require heavy demolition or removal of a complete cabling system • new construction.

Step 1 ___B___

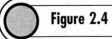

Figure 2.4

INFECTION CONTROL RISK ASSESSMENT
MATRIX OF PRECAUTIONS FOR CONSTRUCTION & RENOVATION (CONT.)

Step 2:
Using the following table, *identify* the **Patient Risk Groups** that will be affected. If more than one risk group will be affected, select the higher risk group:

Low Risk	Medium Risk	High Risk	Highest Risk
• Office areas	• Cardiology • Echocardiography • Endoscopy • Nuclear Medicine • Physical Therapy • Radiology/MRI • Respiratory Therapy	• CCU • Emergency Room • Labor & Delivery • Laboratories (specimen) • Newborn Nursery • Outpatient Surgery • Pediatrics • Pharmacy • Post Anesthesia Care Unit • Surgical Units	• Any area caring for immunocompromised patients • Burn Unit • Cardiac Cath Lab • Central Sterile Supply • Intensive Care Units • Medical Unit • Negative pressure isolation rooms • Oncology • Operating rooms including C-section rooms

Step 2 ___Medium___

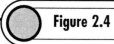

Figure 2.4

INFECTION CONTROL RISK ASSESSMENT
MATRIX OF PRECAUTIONS FOR CONSTRUCTION & RENOVATION (CONT.)

Step 3:

Match the

Patient Risk Group (Low, Medium, High, Highest) with the planned ...

Construction Project Type (A, B, C, D) on the following matrix, to find the ...

Class of Precautions (I, II, III or IV) or level of infection control activities required.

IC Matrix - Class of Precautions: Construction Project by Patient Risk

Construction Project Type

Patient Risk Group	Type A	Type B	Type C	Type D
LOW Risk Group	I	II	II	III/IV
MEDIUM Risk Group	I	II	III	IV
HIGH Risk Group	I	II	III/IV	IV
HIGHEST Risk Group	II	III/IV	III/IV	IV

Note: Infection Control approval will be required when the Construction Activity and Risk Level indicate that Class III or Class IV control procedures are necessary.

Step 3 ___Type B Class II___

Figure 2.4

INFECTION CONTROL RISK ASSESSMENT
MATRIX OF PRECAUTIONS FOR CONSTRUCTION & RENOVATION (CONT.)

Description of Required Infection Control Precautions by Class

	During Construction Project	Upon Completion of Project
Class I	1. Execute work by methods to minimize raising dust from construction operations. 2. Immediately replace a ceiling tile displaced for visual inspection.	
Class II	1. Provide active means to prevent airborne dust from dispersing into atmosphere. 2. Water mist work surfaces to control dust while cutting. 3. Seal unused doors with duct tape. 4. Block off and seal air vents. 5. Place dust mat at entrance and exit of work area. 6. Remove or isolate HVAC system in areas where work is being performed.	1. Wipe work surfaces with disinfectant. 2. Contain construction waste before transport in tightly covered containers. 3. Wet mop and/or vacuum with HEPA filtered vacuum before leaving work area. 4. Remove isolation of HVAC system in areas where work is being performed.
Class III	1. Remove or isolate HVAC system in area where work is being done to prevent contamination of duct system. 2. Complete all critical barriers i.e. sheetrock, plywood, plastic, to seal area from non work area or implement control cube method (cart with plastic covering and sealed connection to work site with HEPA vacuum for vacuuming prior to exit) before construction begins. 3. Maintain negative air pressure within work site utilizing HEPA equipped air filtration units. 4. Contain construction waste before transport in tightly covered containers. 5. Cover transport receptacles or carts. Tape covering unless solid lid.	1. Do not remove barriers from work area until completed project is inspected by the owner's Safety Department and Infection Control Department and thoroughly cleaned by the owner's Environmental Services Department. 2. Remove barrier materials carefully to minimize spreading of dirt and debris associated with construction. 3. Vacuum work area with HEPA filtered vacuums. 4. Wet mop area with disinfectant. 5. Remove isolation of HVAC system in areas where work is being performed.

Figure 2.4 INFECTION CONTROL RISK ASSESSMENT
MATRIX OF PRECAUTIONS FOR CONSTRUCTION & RENOVATION (CONT.)

Description of Required Infection Control Precautions by Class

	During Construction Project	Upon Completion of Project
Class IV	1. Isolate HVAC system in area where work is being done to prevent contamination of duct system. 2. Complete all critical barriers i.e., sheetrock, plywood, plastic, to seal area from non work area or implement control cube method (cart with plastic covering and sealed connection to work site with HEPA vacuum for vacuuming prior to exit) before construction begins. 3. Maintain negative air pressure within work site utilizing HEPA equipped air filtration units. 4. Seal holes, pipes, conduits, and punctures appropriately. 5. Construct anteroom and require all personnel to pass through this room so they can be vacuumed using a HEPA vacuum cleaner before leaving work site or they can wear cloth or paper coveralls that are removed each time they leave the work site. 6. All personnel entering work site are required to wear shoe covers. Shoe covers must be changed each time the worker exits the work area. 7. Do not remove barriers from work area until completed project is inspected by the owner's Safety Department and Infection Control Department and thoroughly cleaned by the owner's Environmental Services Department.	1. Remove barrier material carefully to minimize spreading of dirt and debris associated with construction. 2. Contain construction waste before transport in tightly covered containers. 3. Cover transport receptacles or carts. Tape covering unless solid lid. 4. Vacuum work area with HEPA filtered vacuums. 5. Wet mop area with disinfectant. 6. Remove isolation of HVAC system in areas where work is being performed.

Step 4:

Identify the areas surrounding the project area, assessing potential impact.

Unit Below	Unit Above	Lateral	Behind	Front
		Medium		**Medium**
Risk Group	Risk Group	Risk Group	Risk Group	Risk Group

Figure 2.4

INFECTION CONTROL RISK ASSESSMENT
MATRIX OF PRECAUTIONS FOR CONSTRUCTION & RENOVATION (CONT.)

Step 5:
Identify specific site of activity e.g., patient rooms, medication room, etc. __Office Area__

Step 6:
Identify issues related to: ventilation, plumbing, electrical in terms of the occurrence of probable outages.

Step 7:
Identify containment measures, using prior assessment.
What types of barriers? (E.g., solids wall barriers); Will HEPA filtration be required?
__Barrier at nurses station, walk of mats, cover vents, dust control, covered trash__

_____

(Note: Renovation/construction area shall be isolated from the occupied areas during construction and shall be negative with respect to surrounding areas).

Step 8:
Consider potential risk of water damage. Is there a risk due to compromising structural integrity?
(eg, wall, ceiling, roof) __n/a__

Step 9:
Work hours: Can or will the work be done during non-patient care hours? __n/a__

Step 10:
Do plans allow for adequate number of isolation/negative airflow rooms? __n/a__

Step 11:
Do the plans allow for the required number & type of handwashing sinks? __n/a__

Step 12:
Does the infection control staff agree with the minimum number of sinks for this project?
(Verify against AIA Guidelines for types and area) __n/a__

Step 13:
Does the infection control staff agree with the plans relative to clean and soiled utility rooms? __n/a__

Step 14:
Plan to discuss the following containment issues with the project team
e.g., traffic flow, housekeeping, debris removal (how and when) _____

Plan to discuss the following containment issues with the project team (e.g., traffic flow, housekeeping, debris removal [how and when]).

Figure 2.5

ADMINISTRATIVE, ENVIRONMENTAL, AND RESPIRATORY-PROTECTION CONTROLS FOR SELECTED HEALTHCARE SETTINGS**

This model worksheet should be considered for use in performing TB risk assessments for health-care settings and nontraditional facility-based settings. Facilities with more than one type of setting will need to apply this table to each setting.

Scoring: ✓ or Y = Yes X or N = No NA = Not Applicable

1. Incidence of TB

a. What is the incidence of TB in your community (county or region served by the health-care setting), and how does it compare with the state and national average? (Incidence is the number of TB cases in your community during the previous year. A rate of TB cases per 100,000 persons should be obtained for comparison.)* This information can be obtained from the state or local health department.

Community _____ State _____ National _____

b. What is the incidence of TB in your facility and specific settings, and how do those rates compare?

Facility _____ Dept. 1 _____ Dept. 2 _____ Dept. 3 _____

c. Are patients with suspected or confirmed TB disease encountered in your setting (inpatient and outpatient)? _____

1) If yes, how many are treated in your health-care setting in 1 year? (Review laboratory data, infection-control records, and databases containing discharge diagnoses for this information.)

	Suspected	Confirmed
1 year ago	_____	_____
2 years ago	_____	_____
5 years ago	_____	_____

2) If no, does your health-care setting have a plan for the triage of patients with suspected or confirmed TB disease? _____

d. Currently, does your health-care setting have a cluster of persons with confirmed TB disease that might be a result of ongoing transmission of *Mycobacterium tuberculosis*? _____

2. Risk classification

a. Inpatient settings
1) How many inpatient beds are in your inpatient setting?_____
2) How many patients with TB disease are encountered in the inpatient setting in 1 year? (Review laboratory data, infection-control records, and databases containing discharge diagnoses.) _____

Previous year _____   Five years ago _____

---

* If the population served by the health-care facility is not representative of the community in which the facility is located, an alternate comparison population might be appropriate.

** (Source: Guidelines for preventing the transmission of Mycobacterium tuberculosis in Health-Care Settings, 2005. Appendix B.)

Figure 2.5 | ADMINISTRATIVE, ENVIRONMENTAL, AND RESPIRATORY-PROTECTION CONTROLS FOR SELECTED HEALTHCARE SETTINGS** (CONT.)

3) Depending on the number of beds and TB patients encountered in 1 year, what is the risk classification for your inpatient setting?

Low _____   Medium_____   Potential ongoing transmission _____

4) Does your health-care setting have a plan for triaging patients with suspected or confirmed TB disease? _____

b. Outpatient settings
  1) How many TB patients are evaluated at your outpatient setting in 1 year? (Review laboratory data, infection-control records, and databases containing discharge diagnoses for this information.) _____

  Previous year _____   Five years ago _____

  2) Is your health-care setting a TB clinic? (If yes, a classification of at least medium risk is recommended.) _____

  3) Does evidence exist that a high incidence of TB disease has been observed in the community that the health-care setting serves? _____

  4) Does evidence exist of person-to-person transmission in the health-care setting? (Use information from case reports. Determine if any TST or blood assay for M. tuberculosis [BAMT] conversions have occurred among health-care workers [HCWs].) _____

  5) Does evidence exist that ongoing or unresolved health-care-associated transmission has occurred in the health-care setting (based on case reports)?_____

  6) Does a high incidence of immunocompromised patients or HCWs in the health-care setting exist? _____

  7) Have patients with drug-resistant TB disease been encountered in your health-care setting within the previous 5 years? _____

  Year encountered   _____

  8) When was the first time a risk classification was done for your health-care setting? _____

  Date of classification   _____

  9) Considering the items above, would your health-care setting need a higher risk classification? _____

  10) Depending on the number of TB patients evaluated in 1 year, what is the risk classification for your outpatient setting (see Appendix C)?

  Low _____   Medium_____   Potential ongoing transmission _____

  11) Does your health-care setting have a plan for the triage of patients with suspected or confirmed TB disease? _____

c. Nontraditional facility-based settings
  1) How many TB patients are encountered at your setting in 1 year? _____

  Previous year _____   5 years ago _____

Figure 2.5 | **ADMINISTRATIVE, ENVIRONMENTAL, AND RESPIRATORY-PROTECTION CONTROLS FOR SELECTED HEALTHCARE SETTINGS**** (CONT.)

2) Does evidence exist that a high incidence of TB disease has been observed in the community that the setting serves? _____

3) Does evidence exist of person-to-person transmission in the setting? _____

4) Have any recent TST or BAMT conversions occurred among staff or clients?

5) Is there a high incidence or prevalence of immunocompromised patients or HCWs in the setting? _____

6) Have patients with drug-resistant TB disease been encountered in your health-care setting within the previous 5 years? _____

   Year encountered _____

7) When was the first time a risk classification was done for your setting?

   Date of classification _____

8) Considering the items above, would your setting require a higher risk classification? _____

9) Does your setting have a plan for the triage of patients with suspected or confirmed TB disease? _____

10) Depending on the number of patients with TB disease who are encountered in a nontraditional setting in 1 year, what is the risk classification for your setting (see Appendix C)?

   Low _____   Medium_____   Potential ongoing transmission _____

3. Screening of HCWs for *M. tuberculosis* infection
   a. Does the health-care setting have a TB screening program for HCWs? _____
      If yes, which HCWs are included in the TB screening program? (check all that apply)

   ____ Physicians
   ____ Mid-level practitioners
        (nurse practitioners [NP] and
        physician assistants [PA])
   ____ Nurses
   ____ Administrators
   ____ Laboratory workers
   ____ Respiratory therapists
   ____ Physical therapists
   ____ Contract staff
   ____ Construction or renovation workers

   ____ Service workers
   ____ Janitorial staff
   ____ Maintenance or engineering staff
   ____ Transportation staff
   ____ Dietary staff
   ____ Receptionists
   ____ Trainees and students
   ____ Volunteers
   ____ Others _____

   b. Is baseline skin testing performed with two-step TST for HCWs? _____

       Infection Control Program Guide

Figure 2.5 — **ADMINISTRATIVE, ENVIRONMENTAL, AND RESPIRATORY-PROTECTION CONTROLS FOR SELECTED HEALTHCARE SETTINGS**** (CONT.)

c. Is baseline testing performed with QuantiFERON®-TB or other BAMT for HCWs? _____

d. How frequently are HCWs tested for *M. tuberculosis* infection?

Frequency _____

e. Are *M. tuberculosis* infection test records maintained for HCWs? _____

f. Where are test records for HCWs maintained?

Location _____

g. Who maintains the records?

Name _____

h. If the setting has a serial TB screening program for HCWs to test for *M. tuberculosis* infection, what are the conversion rates for the previous years?[†]

1 year ago _____ 2 years ago _____ 3 years ago _____

4 years ago _____ 5 years ago _____

i. Has the test conversion rate for *M. tuberculosis* infection been increasing or decreasing, or has it remained the same over the previous 5 years? (check one)

____ Increasing ____ Decreasing ____ No change in previous 5 years

j. Do any areas of the health-care setting (e.g., waiting rooms or clinics) or any group of HCWs (e.g., laboratory workers, emergency department staff, respiratory therapists, and HCWs who attend bronchoscopies) have a test conversion rate for *M. tuberculosis* infection that exceeds the health-care setting's annual average? _____
If yes, list.

_____
_____
_____
_____
_____
_____
_____
_____

† Test conversion rate is calculated by dividing the number of conversions among HCWs by the number of HCWs who had previous negative results during a certain period (see Supplement, Surveillance and Detection of *M. tuberculosis* infections in Health-Care Settings).

Figure 2.5 ADMINISTRATIVE, ENVIRONMENTAL, AND RESPIRATORY-PROTECTION CONTROLS FOR SELECTED HEALTHCARE SETTINGS** (CONT.)

k. For HCWs who have positive test results for *M. tuberculosis* infection and who leave employment at the health setting, are efforts made to communicate test results and recommend follow-up of latent TB infection treatment with the local health department or their primary physician?

4. TB Infection-control program

a. Does the health-care setting have a written TB infection-control plan? _____

b. Who is responsible for the infection-control program? _____

c. When was the TB infection-control plan first written? _____

d. When was the TB infection-control plan last reviewed or updated? _____

e. Does the written infection-control plan need to be updated based on the timing of the previous update (i.e., >1 year, changing TB epidemiology of the community or setting, the occurrence of a TB outbreak, change in state or local TB policy, or other factors related to a change in risk for transmission of *M. tuberculosis*)?

f. Does the health-care setting have an infection-control committee (or another committee with infection-control responsibilities)?

   1) If yes, which groups are represented on the infection-control committee? (check all that apply)

___Physicians	___Health and safety staff
___Nurses	___Administrator
___Epidemiologists	___Risk assessment
___Engineers	___Quality control
___Pharmacists	___Others (specify)
___Laboratory personnel	

   2) If no, what committee is responsible for infection control in the setting?

   Committee _____

5. Implementation of TB infection-control plan based on review by infection-control committee

a. Has a person been designated to be responsible for implementing an infection-control plan in your health-care setting? _____

   If yes, list the name. _____

b. Based on a review of the medical records, what is the average number of days for the following:
   ___ Presentation of patient until collection of specimen.
   ___ Specimen collection until receipt by laboratory.
   ___ Receipt of specimen by laboratory until smear results are provided to health-care provider.

| Figure 2.5 | ADMINISTRATIVE, ENVIRONMENTAL, AND RESPIRATORY-PROTECTION CONTROLS FOR SELECTED HEALTHCARE SETTINGS** (CONT.) |

_____ Diagnosis until initiation of standard antituberculosis treatment.

_____ Receipt of specimen by laboratory until culture results are provided to health-care provider.

_____ Receipt of specimen by laboratory until drug-susceptibility results are provided to health-care provider.

_____ Receipt of drug-susceptibility results until adjustment of antituberculosis treatment, if indicated.

_____ Admission of patient to hospital until placement in airborne infection isolation (AII).

c. Through what means (e.g., review of TST or BAMT conversion rates, patient medical records, and time analysis) are lapses in infection control recognized?

Means _____

_____

d. What mechanisms are in place to correct lapses in infection control?

Mechanisms _____

_____

e. Based on measurement in routine QC exercises, is the infection-control plan being properly implemented? _____

f. Is ongoing training and education regarding TB infection-control practices provided for HCWs? _____

6. Laboratory processing of TB-related specimens, tests, and results based on laboratory review

a. Which of the following tests are either conducted in-house at your health-care setting's laboratory or sent out to a reference laboratory? (check all that apply)

In-house	Sent out	
_____	_____	Acid-fast bacilli (AFB) smears
_____	_____	Culture using liquid media (e.g., Bactec and MB-BacT)
_____	_____	Culture using solid media
_____	_____	Drug-susceptibility testing
_____	_____	Nucleic acid amplification testing

b. What is the usual transport time for specimens to reach the laboratory for the following tests?

AFB smears _____

Culture using liquid media (e.g., Bactec, MB-BacT) _____

Culture using solid media _____

> **Figure 2.5** **ADMINISTRATIVE, ENVIRONMENTAL, AND RESPIRATORY-PROTECTION CONTROLS FOR SELECTED HEALTHCARE SETTINGS**** (CONT.)

Drug-susceptibility testing _____

Nucleic acid amplification testing _____

Other (specify) _____

c. Does the laboratory at your health-care setting or the reference laboratory used by your health-care setting report AFB smear results for all patients within 24 hours of receipt of specimen? What is the procedure for weekends?

7. Environmental controls

a. Which environmental controls are in place in your health-care setting? (check all that apply and describe)

Environmental control	**Description**
_____ All rooms	_____
_____ Local exhaust ventilation (enclosing devices and exterior devices)	_____
_____ General ventilation (e.g., single-pass system, recirculation system)	_____
_____ Air-cleaning methods (e.g., high efficiency particulate air [HEPA] filtration and ultraviolet germicidal irradiation [UVGI])	_____

b. What are the actual air changes per hour (ACH) and design for various rooms in the setting?

Room	**ACH**	**Design**
_____	_____	_____
_____	_____	_____
_____	_____	_____
_____	_____	_____
_____	_____	_____

Figure 2.5 ADMINISTRATIVE, ENVIRONMENTAL, AND RESPIRATORY-PROTECTION CONTROLS FOR SELECTED HEALTHCARE SETTINGS** (CONT.)

c. Which of the following local exterior or enclosing devices such as exhaust ventilation devices are used in your health-care setting? (check all that apply)

____ Laboratory hoods

____ Booths for sputum induction

____ Tents or hoods for enclosing patient or procedure

d. What general ventilation systems are used in your health-care setting? (check all that apply)

____ Single-pass system

____ Variable air volume

____ Constant air volume

____ Recirculation system

____ Other (specify)_____

e. What air-cleaning methods are used in your health-care setting? (check all that apply)

HEPA filtration

____ Fixed room-air recirculation systems

____ Portable room-air recirculation systems

UVGI

____ Duct irradiation

____ Upper-air irradiation

____ Portable room-air cleaners

f. How many AII rooms are in the health-care setting?

Quantity _____

g. What ventilation methods are used for AII rooms? (check all that apply)

Primary: (general ventilation)

____ Single-pass heating, ventilating, and air conditioning (HVAC)

____ Recirculating HVAC systems

Secondary (methods to increase equivalent ACH):

____ Fixed room recirculating units

____ HEPA filtration

____ UVGI

____ Other

(specify)_____

Figure 2.5 **ADMINISTRATIVE, ENVIRONMENTAL, AND RESPIRATORY-PROTECTION CONTROLS FOR SELECTED HEALTHCARE SETTINGS** ** (CONT.)

h. Does your health-care setting employ, have access to, or collaborate with an environmental engineer (e.g., professional engineer) or other professional with appropriate expertise (e.g., certified industrial hygienist) for consultation on design specifications, installation, maintenance, and evaluation of environmental controls? _____

i. Are environmental controls regularly checked and maintained with results recorded in maintenance logs? _____

j. Is the directional airflow in All rooms checked daily when in use with smoke tubes or visual checks? _____

k. Are these results readily available? _____

l. What procedures are in place if the All room pressure is not negative? _____
    _____
    _____

m. Do All rooms meet the recommended pressure differential of 0.01-inch water column negative to surrounding structures? _____

8. Respiratory-protection program

a. Does your health-care setting have a written respiratory-protection program? _____

b. Which HCWs are included in the respiratory-protection program?
    (check all that apply)

    ___ Physicians   ___ Construction or renovation staff
    ___ Mid-level practitioners (NPs and PAs)   ___ Janitorial staff
    ___ Nurses   ___ Maintenance or engineering staff
    ___ Administrators   ___ Transportation staff
    ___ Laboratory personnel   ___ Dietary staff
    ___ Contract staff   ___ Students
    ___ Service personnel   ___ Others (specify) _____

c. Are respirators used in this setting for HCWs working with TB patients? If yes, include manufacturer, model, and specific application (e.g., ABC model 1234 for bronchoscopy and DEF model 5678 for routine contact with infectious TB patients).

Manufacturer	Model	Specific application
_____	_____	_____
_____	_____	_____
_____	_____	_____
_____	_____	_____
_____	_____	_____

```
  ●  ┌──────────────┐   ADMINISTRATIVE, ENVIRONMENTAL, AND RESPIRATORY-PROTECTION
     │  Figure 2.5  │   CONTROLS FOR SELECTED HEALTHCARE SETTINGS** (CONT.)
     └──────────────┘
```

d. Is annual respiratory-protection training for HCWs performed by a person with advanced training in respiratory protection? _____

e. Does your health-care setting provide initial fit testing for HCWs? _____

   If yes, when is it conducted?   Date _____

f. Does your health-care setting provide periodic fit testing for HCWs? _____
   If yes, when and how frequently is it conducted?

   Date _____   Frequency _____

g. What method of fit testing is used?

   Method _____

h. Is qualitative fit testing used? _____

i. Is quantitative fit testing used? _____

9. Reassessment of TB risk

a. How frequently is the TB risk assessment conducted or updated in the health-care setting? Frequency _____

b. When was the last TB risk assessment conducted?   Date _____

c. What problems were identified during the previous TB risk assessment?

   1) _____
      _____

   2) _____
      _____

   3) _____
      _____

   4) _____
      _____

   5) _____
      _____

> **Figure 2.5** ADMINISTRATIVE, ENVIRONMENTAL, AND RESPIRATORY-PROTECTION CONTROLS FOR SELECTED HEALTHCARE SETTINGS** (CONT.)

d. What actions were taken to address the problems identified during the previous TB risk assessment?

1) _____

_____

2) _____

_____

3) _____

_____

4) _____

_____

5) _____

_____

e. Did the risk classification need to be revised as a result of the last TB risk assessment?

Preventing and controlling HAIs and identifying risk areas

The Joint Commission's infection control (IC) standard requires organizations to establish priorities and goals for preventing the development of healthcare-associated infections (HAI) within the hospital. These priorities and goals must be based on each hospital's assessed risks. It is the IC committee's (IC) responsibility to prioritize those goals to guide the choice and design of strategies for infection prevention.

In today's healthcare marketplace, we realize that resources are not unlimited. Infection risks continue to expand. That's the reason why an IC program must not only identify risks but also choose the high-volume, high-risk, problem-prone areas in which to place the emphasis.

Overview: The main challenges

Hand hygiene

Hand hygiene would seem to be the simplest measure to take to prevent the spread of infection—however, its basic nature and simplicity are part of the problem in regards to making a difference in practice. Even with the advent of alcohol-based foams for hand hygiene, compliance remains an issue. The noncompliance is often across-the-board and involves visitors and physicians, as well as direct care staff.

Because hand hygiene is part of The Joint Commission's National Patient Safety Goals, facilities are expected to measure compliance, whether by direct observation or other measures, and have that information available to regulatory agencies. If staff are made accountable, with commitment from the administration, compliance can be effected—but the accountability must be from peer to peer, manager to staff, and administration must demonstrate buy-in.

Remember: Direct-care staff are not the only ones who need to comply. Everyone from Social Services to Physician Services must also buy in to the commitment to patient safety by using proper hand hygiene. Visitors and patients are also an important component for patient safety. Patients should be encouraged to speak up and let their healthcare personnel know they expect personnel to wash their hands before they touch them.

Speaking up is not enough, however. Administrators, department heads, and frontline staff must be aware of any flaws in the system. In one hospital I know of, the hand-hygiene compliance monitor complained to senior medical staff about the responses by some nurses and doctors to patients who'd asked them if they had washed their hands. Staff had dismissed or in some cases outright ignored their requests. The monitor discovered the situation through interviews with patients.

The Association for Professionals in Infection Control and Epidemiology (APIC), with the support of the Clorox Company, has developed a product known as the Visitor Education Toolkit. This project offers free brochures, posters, and table tents to encourage visitors and families to use effective hand hygiene when in the hospital and to encourage patients to employ good IC measures when discharged. The materials carry the line, "Protect Our Patients." See the brochure at the APIC Web site, *www.apic.org*.

All areas must measure hand-hygiene compliance. The Joint Commission expects to see measurement, using more than one method, in all areas of the facility—including outpatient, home health, laboratory, and nursing services. If The Joint Commission representative witnesses one incidence of noncompliance with a National Patient Safety Goal during a survey, it will mean a Requirement for Improvement (RFI). This was brought home to us during a periodic performance review, during which a surveyor went on visits with home health staff and observed their hand hygiene. Communication between services and disciplines was also a big push. Sharing statistics with employees and visitors can be crucial for an effective program. Posters, graphs, visuals, reminders, and skills fairs can all combine to make everyone aware of the need for scrupulous infection prevention measures of all kinds.

| Figure 3.1 | SAMPLE INFECTION CONTROL ENVIRONMENTAL ROUNDS |

Hospital Name _____

Unit Manager: Complete this form and send to Infection Control by _____ of each week.

Unit_____ **Date** _____

	Yes	No	N/A
1. All Patient food and medication refrigerator temps checked and documented			
2. Glucometers clean			
3. Hand-hygiene compliance (Record number of opportunities for compliance (OP). Record numbers of actual compliance (Comp). Observe at least five people. Record below in denoted column. Use columns to differentiate between nursing, physicians, other disciplines, and volunteers.)			

Nurses/CNAs		Physicians		Allied Health		Others	
OP	**Comp**	**OP**	**Comp**	**OP**	**Comp**	**OP**	**Comp**

Notes: Action plan for each area not in 100% compliance

_____

_____

_____

_____

_____   _____
Signature   Date

NOTE: The Performance Initiative Council requires that departments participate in this process. Thank you for your support.

The human factor

To effect changes in practice, we use a combination of hard and soft science. Hard science is based on surveillance, data management, all the statistics used to back up our practices—those evidence-based procedures. But soft science also has to come into play. The human factor is involved. Healthcare practitioners must be ready to perform a given behavior. We must determine their attitude toward a specific behavior, their belief about how people whose opinion they value perceive the behavior, and their ability to perform the task.

We are taught how to wash our hands by our mothers, again in kindergarten, again in grade school. Once someone has completed school and gone through nursing or med school, they know how to wash their hands. The question is: Do they remember to use good hand hygiene before and after touching every patient? Are they held accountable by their peers, managers, supervisors, and themselves? Would your staff ignore patients' requests. Most people wash their hands when visibly soiled. The trick is convincing everyone to clean their hands before and after entering a patient room, regardless of whether they touched anything in the room, and after taking off gloves—even if their hands don't appear soiled, even if the patient was not touched.

Making alcohol-based products available along with approved lotions and antimicrobial soap will encourage more staff to use appropriate hand hygiene. Alcohol-based rubs reduce bacteria and viruses on hands and are quick and less irritating than soap and water. As you track and monitor hand hygiene, involve employees in the creation of new hand-hygiene policies and in testing and choosing alcohol-based rubs. Most of the time, we concentrate the hand-hygiene program on nurses and physicians, but don't forget the ancillary staff, such as housekeepers, lab technicians, and patient-transport crews, among others.

We can put in place safety devices to protect employees from bloodborne pathogen exposure, but if they are not used, the devices are not effective. To elicit change, those whom you wish to change their behaviors must perceive a risk to themselves or others, that the risk is severe, and the need to make that change. Once again, education and statistics are key to fostering buy-in from all the key players. Infection prevention measures will not progress without your being able to influence decision-makers to support the efforts and to persuade healthcare teams to adopt safe behaviors.

Employee health

One of the large elements in preventing the spread of HAIs is the effectiveness of the employee health component of your IC program. Employee health is strongly involved in your bloodborne pathogens plan, in the plan to prevent exposure to tuberculosis, and in surveillance of healthcare employees. Employee health also has a stake in offering vaccines—including the flu and hepatitis B vaccines, as well as others like diphtheria, pertussis, and tetanus. Many of the old diseases like pertussis and diphtheria are reemerging. For example, in 2006, India began dealing with a polio outbreak that spread into parts of Africa.

Once again, employees' perception of a threat is key. You've probably heard employees insist that they "never get the flu" or that if they "take the flu vaccine, [they] always get the flu."

Personal protective equipment

As with hand hygiene, employees often become careless with the use, or lack of use, of personal protective equipment such as gloves and gowns, masks and goggles. There is no way to remind staff too often of the importance of protecting themselves with PPEs and protecting patients by using the appropriate PPE when caring for any patient. If everyone used the appropriate PPE for any and all patients, against any potential contact with blood or body fluid of any kind, almost no other isolation would be needed to prevent the spread of disease, especially if the employee practiced proper hand hygiene.

Staff training and education
The infection control practitioner's role changes on an hour-to-hour basis, from data management, to construction risk assessment, to making environmental rounds. Being out on the units to make rounds and look for safety issues is one of the best tools the practitioner can use to assess everything from safety to compliance. But always remember that the name of the game is teamwork. Delegate tasks. Enlist the help of the safety committee and anyone else you can with rounds. If you elect to conduct weekly rounds, you are only one person and cannot be on every unit every day. Spread the joy so that everyone takes responsibility for infection prevention and patient safety.

Don't try to look at everything at one time. Pick the area where you are at most risk. One hospital I know had a glucometer with blood on it found during a state survey of the long-term care unit. Glucometer cleanliness became a focus of rounds. Our hospital used to have an issue with under-the-sink storage of everything from gowns to diapers. With that area becoming a priority focus area for us, units became tired of being written up for that offense and now we rarely see any undersink storage of any kind. That can go to the bottom of the list.

Staff apathy, boredom

Employees begin to tune out references to hand hygiene since it is such a high-focus area and so visible. The employee reaction may be "We know that already. Stop telling us." But when practice doesn't bear out knowledge, we have to find creative ways to remind staff. When planning signage, change signs on a routine basis. Once we've seen a sign or poster for a week or two, it becomes invisible.

Education of patients and family is every bit as important. Our facility has large signs up at every entrance reminding families and visitors to use hand hygiene. We have alcohol foam at every entrance and in waiting rooms in ED and Radiology as well as Admitting and the Surgical Care waiting room. Reminding patients that it is "OK to Ask" is just as important. Patients have to understand and receive permission to be their own advocates by insisting that healthcare providers wash their hands when entering their rooms. Patients often fear retaliation if they ask. The facility has an obligation to assure the patient that healthcare professionals want to be reminded to wash their hands and that their safety is our primary concern.

The secret: Hit their heartstrings

You must help employees understand that they are not only protecting themselves by receiving vaccines, but they are protecting the most vulnerable among their patients—infants and immune-compromised populations. Again, one author or one book cannot do everything for you. The ICP with initiative will include seek out and create documents based on the TB control plan, bloodborne pathogen plan, etc., and tailor them to individual facilities.

In addition to promoting employee and patient protection from influenza and other diseases, surveillance of employee illnesses in order to spot clusters of upper respiratory infections or gastrointestinal disturbances can help identify small outbreaks among employees. If you identify a cluster of employee illnesses that appears to originate on the same unit or all involve the same symptoms, it might indicate that a patient has a not-yet-identified syndrome or that the employees were exposed at the same time to a common source, maybe a patient or another employee. Another reason to track attendance is to measure overall incidences of employee illness, present a large push on hand-hygiene compliance, and see whether absences go down with greater hand-hygiene compliance.

Elements of surveillance

When you look at overall surveillance for your IC program, don't forget to use your risk assessment. Because you based that assessment on disease occurrences in your community, disease prevalence in your state, and the population and geographic location in your area, you should have a good idea of where the greatest risks lie.

If your hospital doesn't have obstetrical services, your surveillance might not include surgical site infections in C-sections; however, central line–related septicemia in your transplant unit could be a big issue. Most hospital surveillance for infection prevention will include that which is specific to your own hospital as well as surveillance that is required by regulatory agencies.

Your surveillance program will most likely include monitoring for ventilator-associated pneumonia (VAP) and central line–related bloodstream infections (CBSI). You will look at resistant *Staph aureus*, strep, and *enterococcus*. But you might also follow Foley-related urinary tract infections in your long-term care unit UAC-related septicemias (i.e., umbilical arterial catheter) in the neonatal intensive care unit (NICU).

Surgical infection surveillance will depend on the type of surgeries your facility performs. Joint implants and gastroplastic, and coronary artery bypass graft surgeries are often tracked, as are colon and cardiac surgeries and hysterectomies.

Once again, *monitoring high-risk, high-volume, and problem-prone procedures is critical.* The surgical specialties performed most often, those at highest risk for complications, or those that have experienced clusters of infections in the past would be the areas in which to begin. When you examine one area and no significant findings occur, end surveillance of that area in order to include a new area that might need attention.

When looking at data, benchmark against National Nosocomial Infection Surveillance (NNIS) data, your own facility data for past years (you might want to further drill this down to timelines with those at your facility who compile this data), and data from hospitals that are similar to yours. Watch for spikes as well as trends. When you see a spike, do the usual investigation, looking for common elements such as physician, organism, or risk factors. Then if the spike continues, look again—even deeper, especially at processes such as whether every staff member performs abdominal preps the same way or whether the C-section rooms are cleaned the same as the operating rooms.

Because the NNIS data is based upon rates, such as # *infections divided by number of surgeries that month* x 100, calculate your data with similar rates. While looking at rates, also consider breaking cases out according to risk factors, such as American Society of Anesthesiologists scores, length of surgery case, wound classification (e.g., class I—clean, class II—clean contaminated, class III—contaminated, class IV—dirty). Further stratification may be used in the NICU by birth weight, or by subtracting 1 from the number of risk factors noted when the procedure was done with the assistance of a laparoscope.

Surveillance and resident pathology

In addition to surgical procedures, pay attention to device use and any related infections. Following infections related to Foley catheters, central lines, ventilators, or other devices is as crucial as following procedures like joint replacements. Resistant-organism trends can show if instances of community-acquired organisms are increasing, especially methicillin-resistant *Staphylococcus aureus* (MRSA), vancomycin-resistant *enterococcus* (VRE), C. *diff*, strep. Similar trends may be visible in your HAI rates.

The Centers for Disease Control and Prevention (CDC) guidelines on multidrug-resistant pathogens, which include a more aggressive approach to the controversial issue of active surveillance, were released as this book went to print. Read more about this in Figure 3.2, "CDC releases guidelines to cut drug-resistant infections."

At any rate, the guidelines will allow CDC to respond to critics who have blasted the agency because draft versions of the guidelines did not emphasize active surveillance cultures as recommended by the Society for Healthcare Epidemiology of America (SHEA). SHEA calls for culturing the nares of targeted patients on admission or periodically thereafter to detect and isolate the reservoir of resistant organisms. The SHEA guidelines recommend the practice so patients colonized with MRSA can be placed in contact isolation rather than serving as an undetected reservoir to spread the pathogens to other patients. A 2004 draft of the patient isolation guidelines by the CDC's Healthcare Infection Control Practices Advisory Committee called for more aggressive measures, such as active surveillance, only in the face of ongoing transmission or if prevalence exceeded institutional goals. That language has been toughened up to include active surveillance cultures if the institution is not decreasing MRSA rates or if it has no MRSA and is trying to prevent the pathogen from becoming established.

Many hospitals already do admission cultures and track patients electronically in order to flag their status. If a patient has had MRSA during an admission, the chart is flagged so that, on future admissions, the patient can be screened and placed in isolation until cleared of resistant organisms. On the other hand, some facilities take the position that MRSA is already in the community and that not all patients can be isolated. Their approach is that strict isolation will do more to prevent the spread of resistant organisms than isolation. Evaluate the incidence of resistance organisms in your facility, as well as the cost of routine testing of everyone and more patients in isolation.

Figure 3.2 | **CDC** RELEASES GUIDELINES TO CUT DRUG-RESISTANT INFECTIONS

Recommends five steps

The CDC in November released new guidelines aimed at hospitals and other healthcare facilities reducing drug-resistant infections.

The new guidelines outline strategies to prevent the spread of drug-resistant infections, which are a growing concern in healthcare settings.

The new guidelines seek to halt the rising rates of drug-resistant infections by calling on hospitals and other healthcare facilities to make comprehensive infection control programs a priority and to take aggressive steps to reduce rates of drug resistance, the CDC said in a press release.

During the past 30 years, the proportion of bacteria that are resistant to antibiotics has steeply risen, the CDC said. For instance, methicillin-resistant staph infections (MRSA) are a growing problem in hospitals, nursing homes, and dialysis centers.

The new guidance, *Management of Multidrug-Resistant Organisms in Healthcare Settings*, is available at *www.cdc.gov/ncidod/dhqp/pdf/ar/mdroGuideline2006.pdf.*

"Effective and comprehensive programs to prevent drug-resistant infections are essential to improve patient safety," said Dr. Denise Cardo, director of CDC's Division of Healthcare Quality Promotion in the press release. "Preventing these types of infections requires a constant and concerted effort on the part of healthcare facilities, but it's important they make this a priority. We need to reduce the number of these serious and potentially life-threatening infections-doing so helps patients get healthy and, most importantly, saves lives."
The new guidelines urge hospitals to do the following

- Ensure prevention programs are funded and adequately staffed
- Carefully track infection rates and related data to monitor the impact of prevention efforts
- Ensure that staff use standard infection control practices and follow guidelines regarding the correct use of antibiotics
- Promote best-practices with health education campaigns to increase adherence to established recommendations

Design prevention programs customized to specific settings and local needs

Source: Briefings on Infection Control, *December 2006. (HCPro, Inc.) Available through hcmarketplace.com.*

Isolation precautions: Practice and procedure

Even though the CDC has released new isolation guidelines, the basics will remain in place. In addition to hand hygiene, standard precautions are another one of our most basic weapons against the spread of infection to patients and staff. But staff members often become careless about the basics. For example, you might've seen nurses start an IV without gloves, rip the index finger out of a glove when drawing blood, fail to wear gloves when performing a glucose fingerstick, or fail to clean a glucometer when finished using it. Standard precautions compliance is key for your hospital to control and prevent infections among patients and employees.

One important basic for patient isolation is communication. Everyone must be aware that a patient is in isolation and what kind. Staff don't all need to know what the patient is being isolated for as much as what kind of precautions to use. Even though you feel as though you have educated staff about this area, do it again—and again. I still run into long-time employees who think an AIDS patient has to be in more than standard precautions and has to have a private room. There is no such thing as too much communication or education.

Make it easy for employees to know what kind of isolation to use for which organism. Color-coded charts help, as does placing the IC manual on the intranet for easy access. We use isolation carts that hang on the outside of the doors and allow easy access to personal protective equipment, disposable cuffs, and other isolation equipment. Evaluate your doors to make certain the carts do not impede the doors closing and affect life safety codes.

I cannot stress the importance of continuing isolation education for your staff. They must receive training upon hire, annually, and as often as you feel necessary. If you see an isolation cart without a precaution sign on the door or cart, more education needs to happen. When you have a skills fair, address hand hygiene and isolation with outside-of-the-box presentations, like *Jeopardy!* for IC. Staff not only fluctuate and change continually; they forget anything they don't use on a daily basis. Your birth center may not see MRSA very often, but they will eventually admit that mom with community-acquired MRSA and multiple open wounds that require contact precautions for both Mom and baby.

Communicating with public health

Don't forget that your local state health department can help you with statistics, both national and statewide, for your IC risk assessments, whether TB or general. Each state has its own requirements for reporting and which diseases to report. Make certain you know the ones for which you and your lab are responsible for reporting or sending lab samples.

State health departments often have helpful documents regarding homeland security, disaster plans, and how to handle various disease outbreaks. Also, *www.cdc.gov* and *www.apic.org* are invaluable resources for the IC practitioner, with education available in all areas of infection control and prevention. You will be able to find the CDC's newest TB guidelines on its Web site so you can make certain that you have everything in place after your TB risk assessment is analyzed and you realize you have any changes to initiate.

Detecting and reporting outbreaks

How do you know if you have an outbreak and how do you handle it? The Joint Commission expects you to have a written plan for or at least be able to talk about how you'd handle an outbreak. You must also be able to show, in the IC minutes, the steps you took to control the outbreak and the actions you took to prevent another one. Make sure the entire committee participates and can speak to their roles for effecting change.

The basics of the outline plan include the following:
- Identification of the outbreak(large or small)
- Identification of case criteria (i.e., what makes it a case you would count—remember you already have those kinds of guidelines in place when you look at VAPs or CBSIs)
- Case incidence over a period of time, in graph form, to show the time period, clusters of cases, etc. (e.g., if you compile a line graph, add arrows to it that show actions taken)
- Data collection
- Investigation of the outbreak and factors involved
- Analysis of actions taken to control the outbreak, changes made. and future actions to help prevent further outbreaks

These steps apply for an outbreak of C. *diff* on one unit or an outbreak of influenza affecting the entire facility. Outbreak management isn't new; we've been doing it for years. We simply need to take formal credit for the investigation and analysis. All this information comes to the ICC for analysis and reporting.

Summary: Why the ICRA goes beyond the IC department

In the last chapter I reviewed the details of the ICRA. In this chapter I counsel you to look at management aspects of implementing it. It's amazing how many facets of hospital operations have become part of IC programs and how IC affects hospital operations, from lengths of stay to patient safety goals. The control of infections due to the spread of organisms or mold spores during repairs, renovation, or new construction has become high on the patient safety awareness chart. Something as basic as doing soil samples before initiating groundbreaking when a new part of the facility will be tied into the existing HVAC system can be crucial, but it doesn't always occur to facilities that might be thinking that the groundbreaking is happening outside so it won't affect patients.

The purpose of the IC construction risk assessment is to help prevent outbreaks due to failure of construction entities to employ proper safety measures. IC's responsibility and involvement in these projects does not end with the completion of the risk assessment—it *begins* there. You, with members of your team, must follow up to make sure that the construction and renovation crew follows the guidelines set out in your construction permit. Tasks like using appropriate barriers, creating negative pressure in the work areas, sealing up air vents, and installing walk-off mats are easy for workers to ignore if someone is not on top of it. If you can't keep up with monitoring the construction yourself, then delegate—enlist the help of the safety committee, environment of care services, etc. All aspects of the prevention of HAIs must be a team effort if you are to be successful. Everyone from frontline staff to administration must be involved in keeping patients safe, and no part of the overall picture is more important than the other—except the care of the patient.

Goal prioritization

Working with infection control (IC) issues sets forth many opportunities for setting, meeting, and prioritizing goals. As you prioritize goals, not only will you assess internal goals like your surgical infection rate for cesarean infections, you may also look at various outside agency measures such as those in the Centers for Medicare & Medicaid Services (CMS) core measures, which have several IC sections. All of the goals must be coordinated.

Core measures

In August 2002 the Centers for Disease Control (CDC) and CMS joined together in a project for the prevention of surgical site infections (SSI). They felt if certain measures were undertaken, that 40%–60% of SSIs could be prevented. The primary culprit in many SSI cases appeared to be linked to the over-, under-, or misuse and improper timing of antibiotics. Their goal was to decrease morbidity and mortality of postop infections in the Medicare population by 25%–50%.

Panels of experts were brought together, a list of prophylactic antibiotic recommendations was compiled, and the project was under way. That project has now evolved into the Surgical Care Improvement Project (SCIP). The aim is to prevent surgical deaths and complications and reduce mortality by 25% by 2010, says Dale Bratzler, DO, MPH, Principle Clinical Coordinator, Oklahoma Foundation for Medical Quality Inc. In addition to the prophylactic antibiotic measures, the project has added normothermia, glucose control, and appropriate hair removal to the measures. Other measures include those involving beta blockers for cardiac surgery and venous thrombosis prevention. Review these SCIP measures:

- **SCIP—Inf-1 Prophylactic antibiotic received within one hour prior to surgical incision:** For surgical patients who received prophylactic antibiotics within one hour prior to surgical incision. Patients who received vancomycin or a fluoroquinolone for prophylactic antibiotics should have the antibiotics administered within two hours prior to surgical incision due to the longer infusion time required.

- **SCIP—Inf-2 Prophylactic antibiotic selection for surgical patients:** Surgical patients who received prophylactic antibiotics consistent with current guidelines (specific to each type of surgical procedure).

- **SCIP—Inf-3 Prophylactic antibiotics discontinued within 24 hours after surgery end time:** Surgical patients whose prophylactic antibiotics were discontinued within 24 hours after surgery end time.

Each indicator is stratified in the following manner:

- **SCIP—Inf-4 Cardiac surgery patients with controlled 6 A.M. postoperative serum glucose:** Cardiac surgery patients with controlled 6 A.M. serum glucose (200 mg/dL) on postoperative day one (POD 1) and postoperative day two (POD 2) with surgery end date being postoperative day zero (POD 0).

- **SCIP—Inf-6 Surgery patients with appropriate hair removal:** No hair removal or hair removal with clippers or depilatory is considered appropriate. Shaving is considered inappropriate.

- **SCIP—Inf-7 Colorectal surgery patients with immediate postoperative normothermia:** Colorectal surgery patients with immediate normothermia (96.8° F–100.4° F) within the first hour after leaving the operating room.

Note that critical access hospitals in rural areas may not have to comply with core measures nor submit the results of the measures to CMS. When planning for budgets, account for the software, support, and personnel needed to assist with chart abstraction and data entry. The positive end of this project is your ability to show results as you bring staff and physicians on board and improve numbers. Bringing physicians on board with the project as champions will make it more rewarding.

Once you enter data in the program chosen by your facility for CMS data submission, you will be able to pull an outlier report that will help you see, if a process failed, exactly where. For example, if an antibiotic was not given within the time frame, was it because one physician always fails to order prophylactic antibiotics, or the nurse initiated the antibiotic too soon? Further chart review allows you to drill down to the heart of the matter and improve the process.

Figure 4.1	**CORE MEASURE INDICATORS**

SCIP-#a	Prophylactic antibiotic received within one hour prior to surgical incision — overall rate.
SCIP-#b	Prophylactic antibiotic received within one hour prior to surgical incision — CABG.
SCIP-#c	Prophylactic antibiotic received within one hour prior to surgical incision — cardiac surgery.
SCIP-#d	Prophylactic antibiotic received within one hour prior to surgical incision — hip arthroplasty.
SCIP-#e	Prophylactic antibiotic received within one hour prior to surgical incision — knee arthroplasty.
SCIP-#f	Prophylactic antibiotic received within one hour prior to surgical incision — colon surgery.
SCIP-#g	Prophylactic antibiotic received within one hour prior to surgical incision — hysterectomy.
SCIP-#h	Prophylactic antibiotic received within one hour prior to surgical incision — vascular surgery.

As reports improve, your scores on sites such as Hospital Compare also improve. As you take these results to committees and the executive board, you can demonstrate the increased ability of your medical and nursing staff to collaborate on a project that directly effects your SSI results. See Sample exceptions report and SCIP results reports in this chapter.

The Joint Commission standards

The Joint Commisson has changed its focus over the years from survey preparation to continuous operational improvement. It hopes to remove the frantic "getting ready for survey" mode and instead emphasize being ready at all times for an unannounced survey. In addition to the unannounced survey, the periodic performance review (PPR) is required annually, either performed by the organization itself and submitted electronically or by a visit by surveyors. If the surveyor(s) find requirements for improvement (RFI), you have 45 days following the posting of your organization's accreditation report on the extranet to submit evidence of standards compliance.

For example, a hospital with more than 300 beds would likely have a full survey for five days with three surveyors. For its PPR, we had three surveyors for two days and one surveyor for the third day. During the PPR, the surveyors are extremely consultative and assist you in finding areas that need to be improved before your unannounced survey. The Joint Commission's hospital accreditation standards spell out all the details needed for your accreditation.

If a surveyor finds even one instance of noncompliance with any of the National Patient Safety Goals, it can result in an RFI. If one staff member is observed not using appropriate hand hygiene one time, it could become an RFI. Surveyors will look across the entire continuum.

When looking at hand hygiene as an example, surveyors may check how you measure compliance. You are expected to measure in such a way that you not only ensure hand hygiene on the day shift but in all settings, the same way, so you can be sure that everyone in all settings on all shifts follows the guidelines.

The Joint Commission will also perform an IC tracer. Surveyors may do a tabletop tracer with members of the IC committee. This would follow the scenario of a patient with an infection through the system and evaluates communication throughout the system. For example, the surveyor may ask how radiology is notified that a patient is in isolation and how the chaplain or transporter is notified.

To be ready for an unannounced survey, environmental rounds are critical. All it takes is one set of outdated instruments or a life safety violation with a construction project for IC to receive an RFI.

Performing mock tracers and environmental rounds on a routine basis may be the best way for you to be prepared for your survey. Always make certain that all areas perform IC the same way. If surgery cleans operating rooms a specific way, the birth center should clean the delivery rooms and rooms where a C-section has been performed the same way. Communication is a large piece of what The Joint Commission surveyors will look at, on both the small scale and systemwide.

Be aware of the standards and the changes that happen on a continuous basis. Know them yourself—never take anyone's word about them. You may find that many behaviors will be attributed to surveyors. Something that has been done for years, when asked, may be explained simply as, "The Joint Commission (or the state, or the CDC) says we have to."

So know for yourself what the regulations say. I came across the "penny-in-the-cup" method of refrigerator temperature regulation, wherein a medicine cup is filled with water, frozen, a penny is placed on top. As long as the penny doesn't move, the temperature must be at or below 32° F. I was assured that this method was approved by a Joint Commission surveyor. Always beware of "they said" and "We've always done it that way."

National Patient Safety Goals

As IC programs evolve, patient safety comes more and more to the forefront. National Patient Safety Goal #7 emphasizes the prevention of healthcare-acquired infections by following the CDC guidelines for hand hygiene, investigating any death due to infection, and performing a sample root-cause analysis.

Why are the goals considered to be so important? According to the CDC, more than $5 billion is added to U.S. health costs every year as a result of infections that patients get while hospitalized for other health problems.[1] Patient safety and the prevention of infections must be the primary concern of any infection prevention program.

The Joint Commission surveyors expect to see a culture of safety when they survey a hospital or any acute-care facility. But administrators traditionally look at IC as an issue for clinicians to take care of. If IC and prevention comes to the attention of a hospital executive, it is often in a negative context and expected to be taken care of by clinical personnel. It is rarely seen as a business issue. The hospital administrator often doesn't speak "IC." As IC practitioners, we have wonderful resources for clinical data, but we must translate that into a language understood by everyone.

Making a business case for infection prevention can make your job easier and encourage administration to put more resources at your disposal.

Key resources

CDC

Everything from the hand hygiene guidelines in 2002 to the tuberculosis control guidelines in 2005 to the new multidrug-resistant organism guidelines released in 2006 come from the CDC.

The CDC Web site at *www.cdc.gov* is one of the key sites for continual updated guidelines and new information on outbreaks as they occur. Your state health department is also an invaluable resource for IC issues. Go to both sites often and become familiar with all areas. Both the CDC site and your state health department will have education tools available, including fact sheets for family, staff, and patient education. Unfortunately some of the CDC guidelines are cumbersome—more than 400 pages when printed, with 20 to 30 pages of references. Killer reading but essential to initiate. Finally, the CDC's fundamentals courses will have many of the tools you need to succeed at IC.

Professional Associations

In chapter 1, we recommended you visit APIC's Web site, *www.apic.org*, for everything from certification information to education resources for families and visitors regarding hand hygiene. For IC certification information, visit the Certification Board of Infection Control and Epidemiology (CBIC) site at, *www.cbic.org*. It describes itself as a voluntary autonomous multidisciplinary board that provides direction for and administers the certification process for professionals in infection control and applied epidemiology. CBIC is independent and separate from any other infection control–related organization or association. CBIC is also rich with resources. And don't forget local organizations. One that comes to mind is the Texas Society of Infection Control Practitioners, *www.tcip.org*. Its stated mission is to be recognized as the leading authority in prevention, control, and surveillance of infection control related healthcare issues within Texas, and, to provide affordable educational opportunities to enhance individual and/or team efforts toward infection prevention. Get out and network! When you do, you will surely find valuable resources for education and networking with other IC nurses.

Networking and IC lists are life blood for practitioners. Internet list-servs allow you to keep in touch with other IC practitioners. No matter what your area of the country, you, as an ICP, will be performing multiple jobs and will need the feedback of your peers. Large hospitals often expect the ICP to perform many more functions than one person can comfortably supervise. The smaller facility may expect the ICP to coordinate IC and quality management, as well as risk management. Networking with other ICPs, even if you can't make it to local or national meetings, will help you keep up with new things, find out how everyone else is meeting standards, and will prevent you from reinventing wheels right and left.

Endnotes

1. CDC, "Public health focus: surveillance, prevention, and control of nosocomial infections," MMWR 41, no. 92 (October 23,1992):783–7.

Figure 4.2   CDC HAND HYGIENE

Hospital Logo

Hand Washing

Join in the fight against infection and promote Handwashing

Source:

Guideline for hand hygiene in health-care settings, Morbidity and Mortality Weekly Report 2002;51 (No.RR-16)

Fold In Half

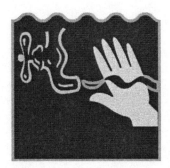

Thank You for Washing Your Hands

Figure 4.2 — CDC HAND HYGIENE (CONT.)

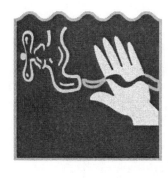

Fold In Half

Thank You for Cleaning Your Hands

Background

Patients are an important member of our healthcare team. To prevent the spread of infection from patient to patient, it is recommended that we all practice hand hygiene.

The best way to do this is to use good hand hygiene techniques. Germs live on your hands and they can be spread when you touch objects or touch other people. Once germs are on the hands, they can enter into the body if you touch your skin that has breaks in it or touch your eyes, nose or mouth. You can spread germs from your hands to other people.

How can we stop germs?

Wash hands with soap water and friction, or use alcohol foam, available in all of our patient rooms.

While in the hospital clean your hands:

- Before eating
- After using the bathroom
- After touching wounds or drainage tubes.
- Before and after touching a patient.

Help your healthcare team by thanking them for washing their hands. If you like, tear off the section to the right and place it on your bedside table.

You are important to the healthcare tam and are encouraged to play an active roll in preventing the spread of germs in the hospital.

Evaluating and redesigning interventions

Along with everything you do is the annual infection control (IC) assessment. Tired of constantly evaluating and reevaluating? Sorry. It's the name of the game, with everything you do in healthcare. You have to look at what you do on a regular basis, change things as needed, and then see how it works. It is the same with IC.

The structure of an evaluation

You and your staff should be evaluating plans and processes on an ongoing basis. You'll want to answer the following questions (after a certain point, these questions should come to you automatically):

- Did our surveillance in one particular area show any problems?
- Should we continue monitoring that particular area?
- Is there another issue that we need to examine more closely?
- Is there one *persistent* problem (e.g., one individual or condition consistently undermining others' efforts or the program)?
- In our evaluation, have we made certain that we have assessed everything we set out to accomplish for the year?
- What changes were made?

The basics of an annual assessment

What The Joint Commission will be searching for come survey time is evidence that your facility formally evaluates and revises goals and programs not only annually but whenever risks change. The evaluation should include changes in the scope of the IC program as new services or sites of service are added. The evaluation should also address any changes in the results of the IC program risk analysis. It must include any emerging or reemerging problems in the healthcare community. For example, to control SARS, healthcare workers in Canada had to change their approach to handling emergency department patients. The evaluation will include the evolution of complying with guidelines based on evidence, successes or failures of interventions, and leadership concerns.

The annual assessment will spell out many of these issues in a simple, easy to look at manner, preferably in as visual a way as possible. Remember that you have to present this information to many medical staff committees, the board, nursing managers, and the rest of the staff. Keep it simple and easy to access. If you go into so much detail that your reader bogs down, you will not be able to communicate with everyone. Communication is key to a good program assessment. See Figure 5.3 at the end of this chapter for the sample form "Year-End Report and Assessment of the Infection Control Program" addressing treatment of MDROs.

When you performed your annual IC risk evaluation, did anything change? Put that in your assessment. Are you going to change your surveillance due to an outbreak, more infections in a specific area, no infections in some area, or concerns by administration or medical staff? Don't forget to include the tuberculosis (TB) assessment because that could affect whether you continue to do annual TB skin tests on all employees.

In your annual evaluation, look at all the interventions you have initiated and whether they are effective. If at the end of one year you can't decide whether something was effective, did you assess it during the year? Any intervention must be checked for effectiveness, whether it is as simple as a new hand-hygiene awareness program or bundling of interventions to prevent ventilator-associated pneumonia (VAP) or flu vaccine coverage. Have you started monitoring core measures? How are your percentages? What kind of interventions have you found effective for improving compliance with the administration of prophylactic antibiotics within an hour of surgery time? What interventions have not improved and how can you change them?

Use your evaluation as a tool to help you obtain any new resources you need for your program as your priorities and focus areas change and evolve. Your evaluation will give you leverage in expanding your department and reaching new goals.

New guidelines

MRSA: All news is old news

As you look at your program, take into consideration the newest guidelines out there. For example, address any changes necessary for your program to comply with the Centers for Disease Control and Prevention's new multidrug-resistant organism guidelines. Discuss the potential for routine methicillin-resistant *Staphylococcus aureus* (MRSA) surveillance with the IC committee and bring to the administration any changes you see in the future of your program.

If, for example, you look at the MRSA guidelines and see the need for continual MRSA surveillance, you will need the involvement of not only administrative leadership, but also medical leadership. For this kind of initiative you would not only be culturing, but also donning barriers and handwashing. Start simple and small and remember that results can be slow to see. Also note that if your facility sees a large population of long-term care patients, that could complicate the results.

Self study is mandatory here. Whether it is part of a formal self-study module or as part of your own independent study, take the initiative and keep yourself up to date. Doing so will allow you to work faster in updating your plan. If you remain disciplined in this task, you may have enough energy leftover to think of creative solutions, or to organize programs to keep staff excited about the topic. See Figure 5.1 for suggestions on self-study.

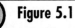

Figure 5.1	SELF-STUDY: THE *CAMH*

It doesn't hurt to get your hands on a copy of the *Comprehensive Accreditation Manual for Hospitals: The Official Handbook*. The *CAMH*, or "Cam," is *the* guide for helping healthcare workers understand the accreditation process as set out by the organization that produces the guide, The Joint Commission. Updated quarterly, the CAMH lists the latest information a hospital needs to improve its operations. The CAMH includes news standards, rationales, elements of performance, scoring, information about National Patient Safety Goals, decision rules, and accreditation policies and procedures.

Among the chapters you'll find in every CAMH are those addressing

- sentinel events
- ethics, rights, and responsibilities
- management of the environment of care
- leadership
- medical staff
- surveillance, prevention, and control of infection

Naturally, you'll want to start with a review of the last item. However, if you can find time to review the entire CAMH—or at least skim the non-IC chapters for IC information—you will find many details that you'll be able to incorporate in your plan. Examples of matters relating to infection control that *aren't* in the IC chapter are those in EC3.10, the chapter relating to hazardous materials and wastes, such as sharps.

At every facility, there is a different keeper of the *CAMH*. Find out who that person is and arrange to borrow it and photocopy relevant sections.

| Figure 5.2 | INFLUENZA: THE JOINT COMMISSION BRINGS LIPS INTO THE IC LOOP |

Under The Joint Commission standard IC.4.15, which took effect January 1, 2007, you are expected to offer immunization against influenza to staff and licensed independent practitioners. That includes not only nursing staff, but anyone who might come into contact with infectious agents (e.g., clerical, dietary, housekeeping, maintenance, volunteers, etc.).

What The Joint Commission will be looking for is a formal program that includes:

- Education regarding the benefits of immunization as well as the health consequences of influenza

- Proof, ensuring that the vaccine is offered annually

- Proof, ensuring that the vaccination is offered at the worksite with interventions designed to increase vaccine acceptance

- Obtaining a declination form from everyone who does not want to be vaccinated

- Monitoring of declination and acceptance rates during flu season and reporting of those rates to administration and units themselves

Use influenza vaccination coverage as one measure of a patient safety quality program.

Business of business: Getting support from the 'C'-suite

Let's begin with the truth: *The financial decision-makers in your facility probably won't listen to you talk about your IC department's needs unless they believe there is a valid patient safety or reimbursement issue that will affect the bottom line.*

As you evaluate, reevaluate, and redesign your program on an annual basis, think about two things:

1. What is important to my *department*?
2. What is important to the *hospital*?

Your ability to find the link between those questions will gauge your success in getting the money you need for staff and training materials. It may greatly affect the status of the IC department in your hospital and your own status within your organization.

Remember that part of your job is to convince administration to put their entire support behind your program. Administration is strongly influenced by regulatory concerns, government requirements, the hospital's organizational board, professional organizations, consumer attitudes, purchaser demands, and third party payers. You know that IC is of paramount importance. However, the people in the cancer ward think the same thing about cancer care, as do the people in pediatrics about child health, etc.—all departments in the hospital. How can you convince your CEO to put the support behind your program that you deserve?

Let's build upon the two points set out above. You need to analyze your organization's priority, for example, in terms of financial health or patient safety, or even both. Then frame your objective to match that priority. It's all about speaking the same language. Explain what the program does well and what you cannot do due to a lack of resources or support of others. Estimate what you need and put it in writing along with a cost estimate with at least three options, knowing you can live with the least of the three options.

For example, if you want to initiate a certain protection and prevention program, or an intervention program, estimate the cost:

- Fact sheets, poster
- Pre- and post-tests
- Self-study module
- Incentives for completion

IC is ultimately a balance between the costs and benefits of the IC program. With the advent of so many unfunded mandates, such as Surgical Care Improvement, (in many cases) mandatory state reporting, and National Patient Safety Goals such as hand-hygiene compliance and sentinel events related to healthcare-associated infections, bloodstream infection (BSI), and VAP bundles, the IC department has to spend a large amount. And for a non–revenue producing department, this can be an issue. Add to that the nonfinancial cost of these initiatives:

- Decreased visibility of IC practitioners (ICP) in patient care areas
- Less time addressing IC concerns (i.e., isolation compliance, hand hygiene)
- Increased time spent reacting to crisis due to less time for proactivity
- Less time devoted to maintaining and monitoring pervious programs
- ICPs being required to do more clerical work to meet mandates

As you present your options for enhancing resources, find an influential advocate who will partner with you to help you get what you need. Plan for success, meet with senior leaders, offer options, and never negotiate for resources during a budget cycle.

As an ICP, your ability to take complex subjects and present them in a way that line staff or administration can understand will be one key to your success. Speaking the language of your audience and telling them what needs to be done for employee and patient safety will lead to a successful IC program. Whatever your goals are for your program, be specific—make then measurable, achievable, realistic, and tied to the priorities of your institution.

ICPs have the continual challenge of influencing without any real authority. We want to convince staff to do the right thing, but unless we have the support of managers, directors, and administration, we often have no way to hold anyone accountable. Sometimes just knowing what is right for the sake of the patient isn't enough to promote adherence to procedures. In this case, the program has to be stepped up to include accountability as well as incentives. A punitive culture may not be the first choice, but positive reinforcement from immediate supervisors can be effective. It can be as simple as giving a handwashing sticker to anyone you see washing their hands.

Find creative solutions to deal with the time crunch we all feel as we try to do more with less. At one point, for example, our quality resource management department had quality specialists doing the minutes for all the medical staff service committees. As core measures and the SCIP have grown, the quality specialists needed to use their expertise on core measure initiatives and the ICP needed to use her expertise for IC rather than simply chart abstraction. Once we presented the problem to the right group of leadership, we found that several nursing administration assistants could divide the time-consuming minutes between them, leaving us to prioritize in other areas.

The prime consideration for your IC program is keeping the program as efficient and meaningful as possible, while finding creative solutions that enable you to meet your goals. As we have all heard more than once, work smarter not harder.

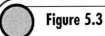

| Figure 5.3 | SELF-STUDY: MDROs |

SAMPLE

Year-End Report and Assessment of the Infection Control Program

Targeted Surveillance for 2005*

Device Related
Central line–related septicemia
Foley-related UTI
Umbilical artery catheter septicemia
Ventilator-related pneumonia

Surgically Related
CABG
Total joint replacement
C-section
Open cholecystectomy

* Gastroplasty surgeries have been added for review in 2006

Surveillance Results for 2005: Healthcare Acquired Infections

Central line infections CCU			
Infection rate per 1,000 device days	2004 = 0.7	2005 = 0.6	NNIS average: 3.7

We've seen a slight decrease in central line–related septicemia and have consistently remained below the NNIS average.

Foley-related UTI_PCC			
Infection rate per 1,000 device days	2004 = 1.0	2005 = 1.0	NNIS average: 3.8

Foley-related infections have remained at a very low rate and continue below the national NNIS average.

Umbilical artery catheter NICU			
Infection rate per 1,000 device days	2004 = 0	2005 = 0	NNIS average: 5.0

We continue to have no umbilical artery catheter–related septicemias in newborns.

Ventilator-associated pneumonia CCU			
Infection rate per 1,000 device days	2004 = 1.9	2005 = 1.8	NNIS average: 6.0

The ventilator-related pneumonias have shown a slight decrease and continue below the NNIS national average

Figure 5.3   SELF-STUDY: MDROS (CONT.)

Joint replacement surgeries			
Infection rate per 1,000 device days	2004 = 2.9	2005 = 2.0	NNIS average: 2.3

Joint replacement infections have seen a decrease this year and are below the NNIS national average overall. We had three individual months with a rate above the NNIS average and those cases were investigated. No actions were required.

C-section			
Infection rate per 1,000 device days	2004 = 0.8	2005 = 2.2	NNIS average: 5.5

C-sections saw several months above the NNIS benchmark, even though the year's average was below. These cases were all investigated and reported to the OB service and infection control. The only trend identified was the weight of the patients. The majority of patients weighed above 250 lbs and some were diabetic. OB reviewed preps, shaving, and patient teaching.

CABG surgeries			
Infection rate per 1,000 device days	2004 = 3.4	2005 = 0.9	NNIS average: 5.5

CABG infections decreased this year and stayed beneath the NNIS average. Preoperative antibiotic use, on time, has increased over the year.

Open choleycystectomies			
Infection rate per 1,000 device days	2004 = 0.7	2005 = 0	NNIS average: 3.2

Infections decreased to zero for this year in open choleycystectomies.

For 2006, we are adding gastroplasty surgical cases due to their risky nature.

- **Overall** resistant isolates are below the national average.

- **Community-acquired MRSA (CA-MRSA)** is increasing all over the country. We are seeing more of it through our emergency room. An inservice on CA-MRSA was presented during the continuing medical education luncheon for the physicians.

- **Nosocomial MRSA** continues to remain steady.

- **VRE** remains constant in both the hospital and community populations

- **C. difficile** appears to be increasing in the community, but our nosocomial incidences have remained close to the same.

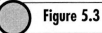

SELF-STUDY: MDROS (CONT.)

- **Sexually transmitted diseases (STD)** continue to be present. However, no new trends have been shown. Reporting is being done appropriately. Chlamydia and gonorrhea are the most common STDs we see in our emergency room. More shigella and salmonella have been noted this year.

- **Hand hygiene** continues to be monitored along with all the National Patient Safety Goals regarding hand hygiene. Our percentage of compliance is at 93% overall with a strong upward trend for the year. It is monitored by direct observation.

- **Continuing education** for hand-hygiene measures continues during orientation as well as the safety fair, Infection Control Week presentations, and Joint Commission on Accreditation of Healthcare Organizations education presentations, and the skills update fair.

- **Flu vaccine education** is an ongoing effort.

- **Risk assessment** did not identify any new areas of concern; however, the addition of bariatric surgery will add gastroplasty review to our surveillance.

- **Education for infection control** has been presented by the infection control nurse. Offerings included housewide educational presentations on hand hygiene as well as articles in the nursing and medical staff newsletters.

- **Surgical site infection prevention (SCIP)** efforts continue as we monitor administration of prophylactic antibiotics one hour before surgery and discontinuing antibiotics within 24 hours.

- We have seen an increase in compliance
  - Joints   Timing 80%–86%   DC 87%–97%
  - Colon   Timing 69%–71%   DC 52%–88%
  - Vascular   Timing 69%–82%   DC 84%–84%
  - Hysterectomy Timing 62%–71%   DC 80%–88%

Physician education will continue in order to further increase our percentages.

Figure 5.3   SELF-STUDY: MDROs (CONT.)

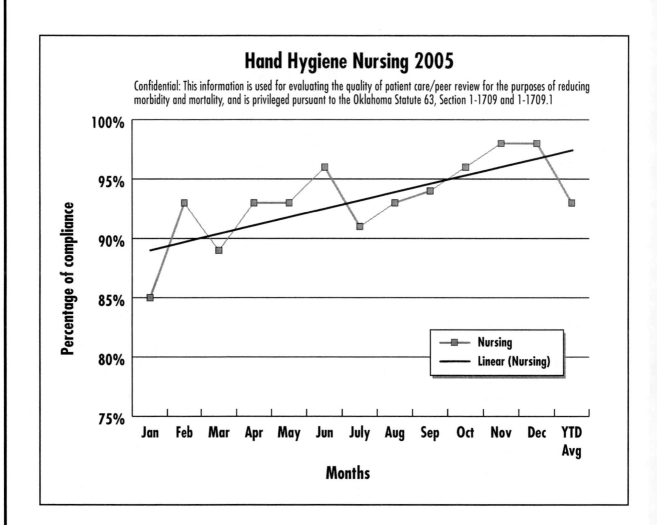

Hand Hygiene Nursing 2005

Confidential: This information is used for evaluating the quality of patient care/peer review for the purposes of reducing morbidity and mortality, and is privileged pursuant to the Oklahoma Statute 63, Section 1-1709 and 1-1709.1

Figure 5.4	SELF-STUDY: THE LAB

When was the last time you met with the laboratory director to discuss infection control? If you have not done so, you should put this on your calendar right away. If the ICP works closely with the lab director, then working together, they may help reduce the risk of healthcare-associated infections. Ask your lab director about molecular typing methods.

What about lab testing? Have you spoken to members of the lab about testing for MRSA, for example? Ask your technologist about mandated screening—what it is, and how it may affect the volume of testing and turnaround times, to name just two of many considerations.

You might also talk about lab safety, like ICPs, laboratorians are very vulnerable to occupation-acquired infections. It is the laboratorian who must send the specimen of the (believed avian flu to the CDC, if need be; it is the laboratorian who must know chapter and verse the latest regulations regarding shipping and transport of infectious specimens.

Laboratory infection control goes beyond best practice, however. Compliance issues involving IC and the lab are another reason for scheduling a meeting with the laboratory personnel. Do you know the latest in OSHA rules on bloodborne pathogens? OSHA recordkeeping?

The Joint Commission and laboratory infection control

The Joint Commission began evaluating hospital laboratory services in 1979. Since 1995, clinical laboratories surveyed using The Joint Commission standards have been deemed to be certifiable under CLIA '88 requirements. Below are items from the 2006 National Patient Safety Goals. Review them with your lab director and discuss how adherence to these goals might fit into your larger IC plan.

#1 Improve the accuracy of patient identification
#1A Use at least two patient identifiers when providing care, treatment, or services.
   Collecting blood samples and other specimens for clinical testing
   Containers used for blood and other specimens are labeled in the presence of the patients
#2 Improve the effectiveness of communication among caregivers
#2A For....reporting of critical test results, verify the complete order or test result by having the person receiving the information record and "read back" the complete order or test result.
#2C ...take action to improve timeliness of reporting, and timeliness of receipt...of critical test results and values

Communication and IC

You might not guess that in reviewing the revenue-cycle side of the lab, Michele Smith, MT(ASCP), CMC, and Dawn Runge, PH, who co-wrote *Lab Billing and Coding: Effective Strategies for Compliance*, would have much to say about infection control. However, maybe not. What they do discuss in detail is the *information chain* leading from the lab to other sections of the hospital and to physician's offices. Their documentation of the types of information

Figure 5.4   SELF-STUDY: THE LAB (CONT.)

failures that can occur has much relevance to IC, if one considers what should happen if an infectious specimen is misplaced.

For more information on shipping and transport of infection specimens, refer to HCPro's *Lab Safety Training Made Simple*, by Terry Jo Gile, MT (ASCP), M.Ed. For more on lab IC, refer to *Laboratory Infection Control: Essential Procedures for Compliance*, edited by Peg Luebbert, MS, MT (ASCP), CIC and Medical Environment Update editor David La Hoda. Each of these books may be ordered by linking to *hcmarketplace.com*.

Disaster

The list of threats our nation faces appears to be endless. We hear daily news about anthrax, small-pox, plague, and Ebola. Then another article appears dealing with chemical threats, not to mention nuclear weapons. Nor can we forget the explosion of the Alfred P. Murrah Building in April 1995 in Oklahoma City or the September 11th Twin Towers tragedy in New York. With this mixed bag of threats, how can we be prepared?

We know there are risks driving to work every day, but we don't just stay home. Instead, we try to mitigate risks by taking action through use of seat belts and air bags. There will always be threats or risks to which we will be regularly exposed. We must choose: Either eliminate threats by not exposing ourselves to them, or mitigate the risks and continue with normal life. I'm in favor of normal life.

With at least two major recent incidents on American soil involving terrorism, both domestic and foreign, disaster management has become a popular topic. However, disasters are not uncommon: 69% of people living in the United States have reported exposure to some traumatic event.[1] A major disaster occurs somewhere in the world almost daily. And disasters and their costs may be increasing. The American Red Cross recently reported that it responded to 70,000 disasters annually.[1] The bombing of the Twin Towers was only one disaster. The Pentagon bombing was another. Add to that the fires, floods, ice storms, and other events happening in the world and you can see why disaster planning and disaster management are so important.

Disaster preparedness: Business as usual, until...

Before the events of 9/11, hospitals had become somewhat complacent. We prepared for the standard things—plans for dealing with fires and electrical failures; in the south, tornado drills are common, in California, medical facilities are prepared for earthquakes. We tend to prepare for the known.

The low probability of a major catastrophe leads to some complacency. We know that the best time to propose major changes for disaster preparedness, including funding, is immediately following a major disaster. When a disaster strikes, the general population expects its public service agencies and other branches of the local, state, or federal government to rapidly mobilize to help the community. We want to preserve life and health. When faced with disaster, medical professionals must be included in all phases of disaster planning as well as immediate response.

...everything changed

The Federal Emergency Management Association (FEMA) considers hospitals to be high on the list for terrorist attacks because the goal of terrorists is to disrupt lives and services and cause as many deaths as possible. So hospitals must be on the alert. Natural disasters are also not respecting of people. A tornado can destroy a hospital as easily as other structures, and hospitals are at risk because of their dependant population.

What's a disaster? Any event that threatens to interrupt business as usual. What would some of the most likely disasters be in your neck of the woods? In Oklahoma, tornadoes are one of the most common natural disasters, with ice storms and flooding coming in second and third, depending upon the part of the state in which you live. In New Orleans, the hurricanes and floods that residents came to expect every year took monstrous forms in 2005, paralyzing the entire area, including all hospitals, business, communication, and emergency services. In Indonesia, earthquake-generated tsunamis are not uncommon. These are all natural disasters that happen despite our best preparations and over which we have little control except for our reaction and any mitigation preparations we've been able to take.

Often, when we think of disasters we think of the large-scale event that can stop a city in its tracks. Since terrorism has been slammed into our consciousness, we, as a nation, are much more attuned to that possibility. Terrorism can manifest itself in many ways and doesn't have to be linked to a political action, or even inner city violence, as we saw in the horrific shootings that occurred in 2006 in Pennsylvania, at a small, one-room school. Such an event, with victims arriving all at once, can more than tax an emergency department (ED).

So why, as infection control (IC) practitioners, are we so interested in disaster planning? Because we are responsible for assisting the safety committee and safety officer in making certain we can handle an influx of potentially contagious patients. And no, that's not just the safety/disaster planner's job. Any disaster has the potential for producing disease, as New Orleans saw with a large number of patients infected by vibrio from contaminated water and with first responders picking up norovirus at refugee camps housing Katrina survivors.

    Infection Control Program Guide

Of even more concern, however, is the potential for an outbreak of a respiratory disease, which could cause the potential influx of hundreds of patients stressing our medical systems, resources, and personnel. We would also have to consider the possibilities of security issues due to panic among staff, families, and visitors. Even worse, if the hospital were under quarantine, would be the people wanting to see their family members inside and those arriving at the ED, just in case they were sick or exposed.

Do you have enough negative-pressure rooms to handle a true outbreak of SARS, avian influenza, or any pandemic influenza? What about a large-scale bioterrorist event with ebola or small pox? The need to vaccinate an impossible number of staff and patients could overwhelm a system, not to mention finding enough staff willing to come to work.

Health experts worldwide are sounding the alarm about new, severe strains of the flu virus, which could result in a rapidly spreading, worldwide epidemic of the flu. According to a Trust for America's Health report, the estimated economic impact of a pandemic flu outbreak today in the United States would be $71.3 billion–$166.5 billion, just from death and lost productivity. The fast spread of diseases such as SARS and H5N1 avian flu across borders and continents has prompted an international conference on infections that don't stay in just one area.

In her June 1, 2005, news release, Karen H. Timmons, chief executive officer for Joint Commission Resources, stated that the prevention of infections from spreading across the world is one of the most critical tasks we face in healthcare today.

In the face of this potential spread of disease, the word *pandemic* is being used frequently. The June 2007 Association for Professionals in Infection Control and Epidemiology (APIC) annual conference features a keynote speaker who is addressing "Avian Flu and Emerging Infections: Preparing for the Next Pandemic."

Why the concern? Andrew T. Pavia, MD, chair of The Infectious Diseases Society of America says that the H5N1 avian virus, for example, is one of the biggest threats to the United States because we have no immunity. The current mortality rate among people with H5N1 is more than 50%. For more on an avian flu plan, see Figure 6.1 and the avian flu fact sheet, Figure 6.2.

Figure 6.1	SAMPLE AVIAN FLU PLAN

Procedure Number: IFC-313
Date: October 2005

Department:	Infection Control
Subject:	Caring for the Avian Flu (H5N1) patient
Definition:	Safely caring for the Avian Flu patient
Purpose:	To prevent spread of potentially infectious agents while caring for the patient
Equipment:	Isolation room with negative pressure and PPEs
Performance Specifications:	All Deaconess Hospital employees
Resource:	"Draft Guidelines for Isolation Precautions;" Federal Register, 2004; 69(113)

Procedure:

1. Place the patient in Airborne, Droplet and Contact Precautions. If a negative pressure room isn't available, use Contact and Droplet Precautions.
2. If an N-95 mask isn't available, use a surgical mask. N-95 is preferable.
3. Protect the mucous membranes with goggles and/or face shield within 3 feet of patients.
4. Keep the patient in isolation 14 days after onset of symptoms or until an alternative diagnosis is established or until diagnostic test results indicate that the patient is not infected with influenza A H5N1 virus. (Human-to-human transmission inefficient and rare but risk of reassortment with human influenza strains and emergence of pandemic strain a serious concern.)

Previously Revised:	Prepared By:	Approved By:
Previously revised	Infection Control	Infection Control Committee

Figure 6.2

FACT SHEET FOR AVIAN FLU

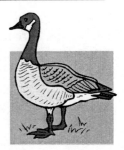

What is avian influenza (bird flu)?
Bird flu is an infection caused by avian (bird) influenza (flu) viruses. These flu viruses occur naturally among birds. Wild birds worldwide carry the viruses in their intestines, but usually do not get sick from them. However, bird flu is very contagious among birds and can make some domesticated birds, including chickens, ducks, and turkeys, very sick and kill them.

Do bird flu viruses infect humans?
Bird flu viruses do not usually infect humans, but more than 100 confirmed cases of human infection with bird flu viruses have occurred since 1997.

What are the symptoms of bird flu in humans?
Symptoms of bird flu in humans have ranged from typical flu-like symptoms (fever, cough, sore throat and muscle aches) to eye infections, pneumonia, severe respiratory diseases (such as acute respiratory distress), and other severe and life-threatening complications. The symptoms of bird flu may depend on which virus caused the infection.

How does bird flu spread?
Infected birds shed flu virus in their saliva, nasal secretions, and feces. Susceptible birds become infected when they have contact with contaminated excretions or surfaces that are contaminated with excretions. It is believed that most cases of bird flu infection in humans have resulted from contact with infected poultry or contaminated surfaces. The spread of avian influenza viruses from one ill person to another has been reported very rarely, and transmission has not been observed to continue beyond one person.

What is the risk to humans from bird flu?
The risk from bird flu is generally low to most people because the viruses occur mainly among birds and do not usually infect humans. However, during an outbreak of bird flu among poultry (domesticated chickens, ducks, turkeys), there is a possible risk to people who have contact with infected birds or surfaces that have been contaminated with excretions from infected birds.

What is an avian influenza A (H5N1) virus?
Influenza A (H5N1) virus – also called "H5N1 virus" – is an influenza A virus subtype that occurs mainly in birds. Like all bird flu viruses, H5N1 virus circulates among birds worldwide, is very contagious among birds, and can be deadly.

Is there a vaccine to protect humans from H5N1 virus?
Currently, there is no commercially available vaccine to protect humans against the H5N1 virus that is being seen in Asia and Europe . However, vaccine development efforts are taking place.

| Figure 6.2 | FACT SHEET FOR AVIAN FLU (CONT.) |

Other things to remember.

- There were no cases of avian flu in the United States or in the Western Hemisphere in 2005 or 2006.

- If we were to have a case, the World Health Organization recommends hand hygiene as the first defense, along with Standard, Contact and Droplet Transmission-Based Precautions, and the use of a negative pressure room and N95 type masks.

- Hoarding Tamiflu is not reasonable because of its extremely short shelf life and the fact that H5N1 has shown resistance to TamiFlu.

For further information visit *www.gov.cdc\flu\avian*.

Internal disasters

An internal disaster is usually small and affects the facility—for example, fire, loss of immediate power, or work place violence. This kind of disaster usually affects a limited number of people and/or patients, as opposed to external disasters such as tornadoes or earthquakes that affect many more. Many disaster plans have elements that cover both internal and external disasters. Anything that threatens to interrupt the performance of essential functions can be a disaster. A gunman running through a hospital's cardiac care unit can stop essential services just as quickly as an earthquake.

Any kind of disaster can occur anywhere, at any time, and can happen to anyone. Start by looking at your facility's structure. You've already assessed your facility and put a disaster plan in place for fire and bomb threats. But have you looked at things like hallways? Do you have unanchored furnishings, unsupported glass interior walls, or obstacles in the hallways? Do your doors function properly? Are storage areas locked? Are chemicals stored appropriately? Plan for survival.

Assessing your facility's risk

From a global perspective, hospitals are in a league of their own in terms of security risks and vulner-abilities. Many people in a healthcare system are unable to care for themselves due to disease or age or mental status. Healthcare facilities include women, children, and infants, a large percentage of our most vulnerable population. Hospitals also contain pharmacies with large amounts of drugs valuable on the street. If the hospital is a teaching or research facility, the possibility exists that they might have to deal with terrorist groups who are violently opposed to animal research. All of these things make healthcare an industry at risk.

Any hospital can be made into a fortress, but then who would come? Every hospital is different and has different populations. People—staff as well as families and visitors—must have access. But this need for access can be a challenge. Some of the most common risks and vulnerabilities in hospitals include

- uncontrolled after-hours access
- uncontrolled access
- environmental security issues
- poor visitation policies and procedures
- inadequate security staffing and deployment
- inadequate security training
- lack of a security management plan
- inadequate security policies and procedures
- inadequate reports and records
- lack of or ineffective security equipment
- inadequate sensitive-area security programs

What makes for a sound security risk assessment?

This is a critical question because standards now require that a facility's security program be as large or small as the risk it faces. There are three issues involved in assessing this risk:

- Who should do the assessment
- How it should be done
- What it should consider

A team approach to the security assessment might include the hospital's existing security staff, members of the safety committee or of a security subcommittee or task force, outside healthcare security personnel, or an outside consultant. Keeping assessment only among facility staff members allows a team approach that can be crucial when implementing the plan.

Because the deployment of security resources hinges on the risk assessment, the format in which the assessment is presented is important. Some options include the checklist approach, the narrative format, or an outside consultant's report. Although the specifics of a security risk assessment would be different at each hospital, it should generally assess the following information:

- The neighborhood, using crime statistics from the local/state police
- Patient population and services offered by the hospital
- Historical security incidents and trends
- Input from the safety and quality improvement committees

Hospitals have to inventory each asset in the hospital as a whole or assets in individual departments, whether they're people, equipment, or materials. Once all assets are identified, look at the type of risks that exist to those assets, such as theft, destruction, fire, attack, etc. Then look at the probability and frequency of those events occurring and the financial ramifications should they happen.

The second phase of this risk assessment is a three-part, hands-on physical assessment. Start with the perimeter of the hospital, looking at the geographic area and the protection of it. Then move to the services offered and the patient and visitor population, progressing to the actual facility itself, the doors, the windows, the alarms, and the structure. Finally, perform an internal assessment of security systems—protocols, incident reporting, and training and education.

What is terrorism?

Terrorism is the use of force or violence against people or property in violation of the criminal laws of the United States for purposes of intimidation, coercion, or ransom. Terrorists often use threats to create fear among the public, to try to convince citizens that their government is powerless to prevent terrorism, and to get immediate publicity for their causes.

The FBI categorizes terrorism in the United States as one of two types: domestic terrorism or international terrorism. Domestic terrorism involves groups or individuals whose terrorist activities are directed at elements of our government or population without foreign direction. International terrorism involves groups or individuals whose terrorist activities are foreign-based/directed by countries or groups outside the United States or whose activities transcend national boundaries.

Cyberterrorism

Cyberterrorism is the premeditated, politically motivated attack against information, computer systems, and computer programs. The type of attacks normally included in cyberterrorism are computer viruses, worms, Trojan horses, hoaxes, Web defacements, domain redirection, computer network penetration to access information, denial and disruption of service, and general sabotage of information and services.

Most healthcare facilities are well stocked with computers and computer and information systems. Each facility must look at their risks. What network connections does your facility have? Are they protected by a firewall or some other type of access control? Who provides the services, and are these services being reviewed and monitored on a regular basis? Can the network vendor or provider help? How can the facility recover in case of attack or failure? What security measures can a facility take to protect their Web site from defacement or information theft?

Also look at backup of critical data—whether it should be encrypted and what recovery plans can be put into place.

Remember the following key things to help protect against cyberterrorism:

- All accounts should have passwords that are unusual and difficult to guess
- Change network configuration when defects become known
- Check with vendors for upgrades and patches and apply security patches when identified
- Audit systems and check logs to help detect and trace an intruder
- If you are ever unsure about the safety of a site or receive suspicious e-mail from an unknown address, don't access it
- Install antivirus software on computers and keep virus definitions up to date

The protection of health information services and critical patient information is essential to any facility and must be included as part of the disaster planning.

Bioterrorism

The threat of biological warfare attack on the United States has received a lot of attention in the media recently, but the threat isn't a new one. Looking to history as an example, during World War II, the Japanese had an aggressive biological weapons program, and during the Cold War, the former Soviet Union built an impressive arsenal of biological weapons that could be mounted on intercontinental ballistic missiles.

These days, with terrorism becoming more common, healthcare agencies have accepted bioterrorism as a realistic threat. In April 1999, APIC, in cooperation with the Centers for Disease Control and Prevention (CDC), offered a reference document for use as a tool to facilitate bioterrorism-readiness plans for individual institutions. For a sample bioterrorism plan, see Figure 6.3.

Figure 6.3

SAMPLE BIOTERRORISM PLAN

Procedure Number: IFC-309
Date: August 2006

Department:	Infection Control
Subject:	Bioterrorism Plan
Definition:	The use of a known biological agent being dispersed within the treatment area of Deaconess Hospital or any patient presenting with a disease that is relatively uncommon and has bioterrorism potential (i.e., pulmonary anthrax, pneumonic plague, smallpox, tularemia)
Purpose:	1. To provide for an effective response to an announced or covert bioterrorism attack 2. To identify and initiate a response to a bioterrorism-related outbreak 3. To determine the extent of the facility's bioterrorism readiness needs 4. To provide education to staff regarding bioterrorism
Equipment:	As appropriate
Performance Specifications:	All Hospital Personnel
Resource:	1. Bioterrorism Readiness Plan: A template for Healthcare Facilities 2. APIC Bioterrorism Task Force 3. CDC Hospital Infections Program Bioterrorism Working Group

Procedure:

In the event of an actual or suspected bioterrorist attack, this Bioterrorism Plan will go into effect in order to prevent or reduce the spread of infection to all other persons.

I. Responsibility

A. The Infection Control Committee, in partnership with local and state health departments, is responsible for developing a hospital specific response plan. Implementation and monitoring of this plan will be incorporated into the implementation and monitoring of the hospitalwide emergency preparedness program.

B. Authorization is given to the Infection Control Committee Chairperson or designee to implement prevention and control measures in the event of an outbreak.

Figure 6.3   **SAMPLE BIOTERRORISM PLAN (CONT.)**

II. Reporting

A. If a bioterrorism event is suspected, the emergency response system will be activated. The command center will notify the proper people. Notification includes:

Hospital Administration Pager
DON
Safety Officer Pager
Infection Control Personnel Pager
Local Emergency Medical Systems
Marketing Pager
Police and Fire Departments
State Health Department
FBI field office
CDC (770)488-7100

III. Detection of a Bioterrorism Attack:

A. Announced Attack:
1. In an announced attack, persons are warned by the potential terrorists that an event has occurred. Notification and preparation should proceed, as per the hospitalwide emergency preparedness plan, until the attack is ruled as a "hoax" by proper authorities.
   a. In a widespread emergency involving mass casualties (or the possibility thereof), the department managers will initiate the call back list:
      1) Personnel will report to the Personnel Pool for assignments.
      2) The medical staff will report to the Chief of Staff for assignments.
   b. Department specific responsibilities are delineated in the Emergency Preparedness plan.
   c. The designation decontamination area will be prepared for use.
   d. A designated area will be assigned for the media in MOB B&C.
   e. At the time of activation of the hospitalwide bioterrorism plan, Security Personnel on duty will lock all hospital exits and entrances with the exception of the emergency entrance. Employees and medical staff will be required to wear name tags or carry cards identifying themselves as employees/medical staff. Only persons with proper identification will be allowed to enter the hospital during this emergency. The emergency department will be locked from the rest of the hospital.
   f. All elective admissions and procedures will be canceled until authorities rule out an actual attack.
   g. Patient/public informational material and home care instructions for the most likely biological agents to be used in an attack will be available in the emergency department or from Infection Control.

Figure 6.3   SAMPLE BIOTERRORISM PLAN (CONT.)

B. Covert Event:
1. Due to the rapid progression to illness and the methods of dissemination of biological agents, prompt identification and response is necessary. Healthcare practitioners should be alerted to the possibility of a bioterrorism attack with the recognition of certain high-risk symptoms and scenarios:
   a. An unusual increase in the number of people seeking care with fever, respiratory, or gastrointestinal complaints;
   b. A rapidly increasing incidence (hours to days) of disease in a normally healthy population;
   c. An unusual pattern to a rapidly emerging endemic disease;
   d. An endemic curve which rises and falls during a short period of time;
   e. Clusters of patients arriving from the same locale;
   f. Large numbers of rapidly fatal cases;
   g. Lower attack rates among people who had been indoors;
   h. Any patient presenting with a disease that is relatively uncommon and has bioterrorism potential (i.e., pulmonary anthrax, pneumonic plague, smallpox, tularemia).

C. Patient Management:
1. As with any patient, Standard Precautions are to be used:
   a. Handwashing.
   b. Gloves used when in contact with blood or body fluids.
   c. Gowns to protect clothing and skin during patient procedures likely to generate splashes.
   d. Face shields or masks and eye protection are worn when splashes may be generated during patient procedures.
   e. Respiratory precautions may also be required when airborne pathogens are suspected.
   f. In large scale events, triage procedures will be necessary following the hospital's emergency preparedness plan and Infection Control Procedures:
      1) Cohorting patients presenting with the same symptoms/syndrome is acceptable.
      2) Routine infection control policies and procedures should be followed for patient placement (negative air flow rooms for air borne agents, restricted access, etc.).
      3) In a scenario of mass respiratory isolation, 2&3 north can be used.
2. Environmental cleaning will follow the principles of Standard Precautions documented in the Infection Control manual.
3. Patient clothing should be removed at the decontamination site (if decontamination is called for) and placed in an impervious bag by staff wearing appropriate personal protective equipment (PPE).
   a. The FBI may request the clothing as evidence in their investigation.
4. Clinical laboratories, pathology, Coroner's Office and mortuaries must all be informed of the potential infectious outbreak prior to submitting specimens for examination or disposal.
   a. Specimen packaging and handling must be coordinated with the local and state health departments and the FBI. A chain of custody document must accompany the specimen from the time of collection. **For specific instructions on specimen transport contact the CDC Emergency Response Office, Bioterrorism Emergency, (770)488-7100.**

Previously Revised:	Prepared By:	Approved By:
2002	Infection Control Committee	Infection Control Committee

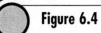

Figure 6.4   SAMPLE PATIENT INFLUX PLAN

Procedure Number: IFC-309A
Date: October 2005

Department:	Infection Control
Subject:	Infectious Patient Influx
Definition:	A large number of infectious patients presenting with any communicable disease (i.e., pulmonary anthrax, pneumonic plague, smallpox, avian flu, SARs)
Purpose:	1. To provide for an effective response to a large influx of communicable patients
Equipment:	As appropriate
Performance Specifications:	All hospital personnel
Resource:	CDC

Procedure:

In the event of a large influx of communicable patients, this plan will go into effect in order to prevent or reduce the spread of infection to all other persons.

I. Responsibility

A. The Infection Control Committee, in partnership with local and state health departments, is responsible for developing a hospital specific response plan. Implementation and monitoring of this plan will be incorporated into the implementation and monitoring of the hospitalwide emergency preparedness program.

B. Authorization is given to the Infection Control Committee Chairperson or designee to implement prevention and control measures in the event of an outbreak.

II. Reporting

A. If a large influx of communicable patient is anticipated, the emergency response system will be activated. The command center will notify the proper people.

Figure 6.4	**SAMPLE PATIENT INFLUX PLAN** (CONT.)

B. Patient Management:
  1. As with any patient, Standard Precautions are to be used:
    a. Handwashing.
    b. Gloves used when in contact with blood or body fluids.
    c. Gowns to protect clothing and skin during patient procedures likely to generate splashes.
    d. Face shields or masks and eye protection are worn when splashes may be generated during patient procedures.
    e. N 95 masks and a negative pressure room will also be required when airborne pathogens are suspected.
    f. In large scale events, triage procedures will be necessary following the hospital's emergency preparedness plan and Infection Control Procedures:
      1) Cohorting patients presenting with the same symptoms/syndrome is acceptable.
      2) Routine infection control policies and procedures should be followed for patient placement (negative air flow rooms for air borne agents, restricted access, etc.).
      3) In a scenario of mass respiratory isolation, such as Avian Flu, 2&3 north can be used. The emergency room will isolate these patients as they are triaged.
  2. Environmental cleaning will follow the principles of Standard Precautions documented in the Infection Control manual.
  3. Patient clothing should be removed at the decontamination site (if decontamination is called for) and placed in an impervious bag by staff wearing appropriate personal protective equipment (PPE).

Clinical laboratories, pathology, Coroner's Office and mortuaries must all be informed of the potential infectious outbreak prior to submitting specimens for testing.

 Infection Control Program Guide

Hospitals and clinics may be the first to recognize and initiate a response to a bioterrorism-related outbreak, so overall disaster plans should address this issue. Individual facilities should determine the extent of their bioterrorism-readiness needs, which may range from notifying local emergency networks (i.e., calling 9-1-1) and transferring affected patients to appropriate acute-care facilities, to activating large, comprehensive communication and management networks.

Although we all understand the need for awareness and education about bioterrorism, your preparation and response can be overwhelmed by the horror of the possible scenarios out there. After seriously thinking about some of the worst scenarios, we all may just want to forget the whole thing and slink away to our beds.

In October and November 2001, the United States suffered numerous casualties due to exposure to a highly lethal strain of B*acillus anthracis* or *anthreas*. Recently, the threat of an attack using smallpox virus resulted in the production of vast stores of smallpox vaccine: enough to vaccinate the entire U.S. population.

Every level of worker should have a clear understanding of the threat posed by bioterrorism and the community or statewide plan to respond. This is crucial so that workers

- will go to work after a biologic attack
- understand that personal protective equipment is available
- know that appropriate antibiotics or vaccines can be delivered from their place of work

Smallpox is generally considered the worst-case pathogen since we stopped vaccinating against it 30 or 40 years ago. However, a bioweapon that aerosolizes the plague bacteria *Yersinia pestis* could create an airborne pneumonic plague. Although antibiotic treatment is possible, the biodefense center reports that 50 kg of *Y. pestis* aerosolized over a city of 5 million would result in 150,000 infections, at least half of which would require hospitalization, and some 36,000 deaths.

Anything contagious would be worrisome in our highly mobile society. Businesspeople travel every day. Before they become symptomatic, they could fly from city to city, country to country, and back, spreading any infectious agent farther than anyone would be able to quickly track it.

Plague and anthrax (B*acillus anthracis*) would be easy to obtain by a terrorist group. The release of 100 kg of anthrax could result in a minimum of 130,000 deaths. In a real-world example, when aerosolized anthrax spores were accidentally released in 1979 from a bioweapons facility in the former Soviet Union, 68 of the 70 people infected died.

Those known or suspected to be exposed to anthrax could end up in long lines waiting for chest x-rays. For people who have a normal chest x-ray, resources would be expended and antibiotics would be used.There is little hope and few medical options for those with evidence of anthrax infection—it's lethal.

While the wild forms of the various bioterrorism pathogens are frightening all on their own, we still must contend with the genetically engineered infectious agents. For example, researchers in Moscow have created a recombinant strain of anthrax, raising the possibility that current vaccine efficacy could be destroyed. With advances in bioengineering, we have the continuing possibility that bioweapons will be created that are resistant to known postexposure treatments and vaccines.

Medical defense against biological warfare is an area of study for military healthcare providers that does not readily apply to the daily mission of caring for patients in peacetime. However, during Operations Desert Shield, when it became obvious that the threat of biological attacks against our soldiers was real, we realized we needed to do more to educate our medical professionals about how to prevent and treat biological warfare casualties. The Secretary of Defense announced in November 1997 that all U.S. military troops will be immunized against anthrax.

Training efforts intensified following the New York City World Trade Center bombing, Tokyo subway sarin gas release, Oklahoma City federal building bombing, and the Atlanta Centennial Park bombing. And the disclosure of a sophisticated offensive biological warfare program in the former Soviet Union reinforced the need for increased training and education.

Dispersement

Many bacteria, fungi, viruses, rickettsial agents, and toxins have been mentioned in literature as possible biological warfare agents. These most often include anthrax, botulinum toxin, plague, staphylococcal enterotoxin B, and Venezuelen equine encephalitis virus.

Despite the different characteristics of these organisms, viruses, and toxins, biological agents used as weapons do have some things in common. The most important characteristic is the ability of the agent to be dispersed in aerosols of article size 1–5 microns, which may remain suspended in certain weather conditions for hours and, if inhaled, will penetrate into distal bronchioles and terminal alveoli of victims. Particles larger than 5 microns would tend to be filtered out in the upper airway.

Differences also must be taken into account because treatment for bacterial agents such as anthrax, cholera, or plague; viruses such as smallpox or Venezuelan equine encephalitis; and biological toxins such as botulinum, ricin, and Staphylococcal Enterotoxin B would all exhibit different symptoms and require varying treatments.

Agents of chemical and bioterrorism

Those organisms suspected of being most likely to be used in an attack, are thought to be anthrax, brucellosis, plague, tularemia, botulinum, and smallpox because they are infectious by aerosols, fairly stable, susceptible to civilians, have high morbidity and mortality, and are difficult to diagnose. Take a look at the following details:

- **Anthrax:** According to the CDC, direct person-to-person spread of anthrax is extremely unlikely. Communicability is not a concern when treating patients with anthrax. That said, every patient should be treated using universal precautions.

- **Botulism:** The gram-positive bacillus Clostridium botulinum causes botulism. Botulism is usually foodborne, however, an inhalation form could be used. The organism produces a potent neurotoxin, which results in a flaccid paralysis that can create respiratory failure and upper airway obstruction. Person-to-person transmission isn't an issue.

- **Plague:** Plague is most often contracted from being bitten by a rodent flea carrying the bacillus *Yersinia pestis* and results in lymphatic and blood infections. The pulmonary variant pneumonic plague can be transmitted person-to-person through respiratory droplets, infecting those who have direct and close contact with an ill patient. For pneumonic plague, droplet precautions should be used in addition to standard precautions. Droplet precautions require caregivers to wear a surgical mask when within 3 ft of the infected patients.

- **Smallpox:** The last cases of naturally occurring smallpox disease were seen in Somalia in 1977. In 1980, the World Health Organization declared smallpox eradicated. In the United States, the practice of vaccinating children ceased in 1972. It is thought that immunity to the disease may have waned and that a booster would be required to speed up the immune response to the disease.

The disease is created by a virus unique to humans and highly contagious after an incubation period. It is transmitted through an infected person's aerosolized saliva droplets or through direct contact with the infected individual's skin when skin pustules or scabs are present. With modern air-handling systems in healthcare buildings, it is possible for airborne transmission of the virus to occur indirectly through the circulating air and heating systems. Airborne and contact precautions must be used in addition to standard precautions when treating infected patients.

Detection and recognition

The likelihood of a biological attack is unknown, and significant defensive preparations are underway; however, what happened with anthrax in October 2001 could potentially be repeated with a worse scenario. The fact remains that humans are often the most sensitive detector of a biological attack. An increased number of patients presenting with signs and symptoms caused by the disseminated disease agent is the most likely first indicator that a bioterrorist attack has occurred.

The CDC created the Epidemic Intelligence Service as early as 1951. This service was created to train epidemiologists in case an attack should take place against the United States during the Cold War. Documenting who is affected, possible routes of exposure, signs and symptoms of disease, and the rapid identification of the causative agents will greatly increase the ability to plan an appropriate medical and public health response.

Many if not most diseases caused by weaponized biological agents present with nonspecific signs and symptoms that could be misinterpreted as naturally occurring. Watching for patterns is an important factor when trying to differentiate between natural and terrorist or warfare attacks. In most naturally occurring epidemics, a gradual rise in disease incidence occurs. People are progressively exposed to an increasing number of patients, vectors, or fomites that spread the pathogen.

In contrast, a biological warfare attack would expose many people at the same time. Even taking into account different incubation periods based on exposure dose and physiological differences, a compressed epidemic curve with a peak in a matter of days or even hours could occur. Response may be based on the recognition of syndromes that should alert healthcare professionals to the possibility of a bioterrorism-related outbreak.

Indicators that might point to a bioterrorism attack could include

- a rapidly increasing disease incidence in a normally healthy population
- an epidemic curve rising and falling in a short period of time
- an unusual increase in people with fever or respiratory symptoms seeking treatment
- an endemic disease emerging quickly at an unusual time
- lower rates among people who had been indoors compared to those outdoors
- clusters of patients arriving from a single locale
- large numbers of rapidly fatal cases
- any patient presenting with an uncommon disease such as pulmonary anthrax, tularemia, or plague

Plans

My goal is to have a one-size-fits-all plan for disasters. Right now, like everyone else, I have boutique plans for every disease out there. I have mentioned that you need plans for SARS, smallpox, pandemic flu, and patient influx (some of which are provided here). I want our disaster plan to be thorough enough to encompass any kind of disaster, outbreak, terrorist attack, or bioterror incident, with an appendix that covers the IC aspect of communicable diseases. If staff have to plow through multiple pages of multiple plans, nothing will happen effectively.

Patient influx

Why has patient influx suddenly entered The Joint Commission radar screen? Two seemingly unrelated words: Katrina, pandemic. With Katrina, hospitals were not prepared for large numbers of patients, lack of communication, utility interruption, and business standstill. The idea of a pandemic without better preparation is enough to put fear into everyone's heart. That's why, as individual hospitals and healthcare centers, we must know how we plan to react to a disaster or patient influx, even more so if the influx contains patients with a communicable disease. For a sample patient-influx plan, see Figure 6.4.

My advice is to make the plan specific but simple and easy to follow. When the emergency is upon you, it's not the time to try and figure out how to comply with a multilayered, complex plan. Everyone must know what his or her responsibility is. It boils down to practice, drills, and education on all levels. All personnel must be involved. Just because you are making plans for infectious patients doesn't mean this simply affects nursing. All staff who have any potential for patient contact must be involved. That might include office staff like admitting, housekeeping, and ancillary staff like lab and phlebotomy, chaplains. Keep an open mind and not only plan for any eventuality, but educate the same way.

If you end up dealing with an infectious disease and the hospital is suddenly quarantined, you will have to make do with whatever category of staff is in the building. During a disaster, you have the potential for other staff to refuse to come or not to be allowed to enter. All of these issues can be addressed in the overall disaster plan, and IC will work closely with the safety director and facilities manager, along with administration, to make certain the infectious aspects are adequately addressed in the disaster plan.

It is essential to have drills for disaster planning, whether full blown or tabletop. Some of these drills must incorporate the potentially infectious aspect of disasters, such as an outbreak of influenza or a bioterrorism event. Working closely with the safety officer and safety committee will allow you to make certain those aspects are not forgotten when drills are scheduled.

Endnotes

1. American Red Cross. "America's Disasters, 2004: Meeting the Challenge." Rockville, MD. 2004.

Data management

An infection control (IC) practitioner (ICP) is typically a registered nurse, physician, epidemiologist, or medical technologist whose goal is to prevent healthcare-acquired infections (HAI) by isolating sources of infections and limiting their spread. You systematically collect, analyze, and interpret health data in order to plan, implement, evaluate, and disseminate appropriate public health practices. You train healthcare staff through instruction and dissemination of information on IC practices.

With the advent of new emerging infectious diseases such as SARS and avian influenza, as well as older foes such as methicillin-resistant *Staphylococcus aureus* (MRSA) and and our old friend, vancomycin-resistant enterococcus (VRE), the role of the ICP is more critical than ever in the age of mandatory reporting of infections. IC and prevention strategies are critical because—as we've mentioned and cannot mention enough—HAIs continue to affect more than 2 million patients annually in the United States, at a cost of more than $5.5 billion. And according to the Association for Professionals in Infection Control and Epidemiology (APIC), control and prevention of HAIs have significantly lowered patient infection risk in hospitals and other healthcare and group facilities, and infection surveillance and data collection on infection rates have become the basis for measuring the quality of care in hospitals.

Certification, regulation, and facilitation

In IC.7.10, The Joint Commission requires the IC program to be managed effectively. What The Joint Commission expects to see is management of the IC program activities by people who are qualified. The required qualifications are determined by the risks entailed in the care, treatment, and services provided, patient populations, and services. The qualifications can by met by ongoing education, training, experience, and certification. The qualified person coordinates all infection prevention and control activities and facilitates ongoing monitoring of the effectiveness of the program.

Continuing education is required by most states and is not difficult to obtain. Many states have annual IC conferences with their local APIC chapters as well as other educational offerings for continuing education credits. APIC has an annual conference as well as education courses for new ICPs to learn basics of epidemiology. Start ahead of time to make sure your education requests make it into the budget early in the year. Remind administration that this is part of The Joint Commission requirements.

Certification is one way to prove the program is run by someone who is qualified because it requires renewal testing on a routine basis. Also, in IC.8.10 The Joint Commission requires allocation of adequate resources to plan and implement the program. Education would be part of those resources.

The Joint Commission is currently in the processing of enhancing, altering, and revising its IC standards. The revised standards reflect increased recognition that HAIs are a national concern and serve to raise awareness that these infections can be acquired in any healthcare setting and increase what is expected of hospital leadership and of IC programs. If you have not done so already, you should be bookmarking The Joint Commission site.

The goal of an effective IC program is to reduce the risk of acquisition and transmission of HAIs. The Joint Commission standards still require that hospitals have organizationwide IC programs, but they also state that hospitals should assign responsibility for managing these programs to individuals formally qualified in IC and epidemiology. According to The Joint Commission Standard IC.7.10: "Qualifications [for the individual(s) responsible for managing the IC program] may be met through… certification [such as that offered by the Certification Board for Infection Control (CBIC)] in prevention and control of infections."

The Joint Commission's endorsement of certification through CBIC serves as an incentive for ICPs to become certified and and maintain their certification. Endorsement of CBIC certification by The Joint Commission also provides the impetus for healthcare institutions to require certification for individuals responsible for managing their IC programs.

In addition to education, other resources include adequate systems to access information for and to support infection prevention—computers, data-tracking systems, lab support, equipment, and supplies. The way to ensure that this happens is to establish an effective program, prove to administration that you are doing the right things, and that you could do things even better with more resources. By continuing an effective program and reevaluating on a regular schedule, you will be able to prove that you save the hospital money by giving the best care for the patients and protecting them from infection.

Risk management

With the rise of MRSA and increasing media awareness of HAIs as well as The Joint Commission's emphasis on the National Patient Safety Goals and prevention of infection, the IC program is extremely visible. The good thing is this gives you more chances to beef up your program. The bad thing is that this gives lawyers an opening to focus on infections.

As patients become more savvy and ask frequent questions, infections, especially HAIs, are pushed to the front of everyone's awareness. We used to assume that some infections are unavoidable, but now we know a lot of those unavoidable infections can be prevented. When you prevent infections, your IC program becomes a profit center because the infections erode hospital profits with increased length of stay.

Infection prevention has become a target as transparency increases and infection reporting becomes public. The compelling evidence that most infections are preventable is a trial lawyer's best tool. Even if there is no evidence that a hospital overlooked standard infection precautions, the attorney could argue that infection is evidence enough that the hospital was negligent. The hospital then has to assume the burden of proving that something other than negligence could cause the infection. Maybe the patient came in colonized with the same organism that caused the infection or had the organism already, just at another site. If the patient aspirated, the organism could have come from the gastrointestinal site.

Following the same standard of care as the community and nation will be paramount. Policies and actual practice must reflect the current state of infection prevention science. Be sure your practice meets policy and that your policies aren't outdated or not adhered to. The Centers for Disease Control has moved to a zero-tolerance approach for infections. That doesn't mean an infection will never happen, but it does mean that when one happens, you will be able to speak to it and ensure that all appropriate preventive measures are taken, including Ventilator-associated pneumonia (VAP) bundling, the use of full sterile techniques during central line insertion, and all of the core measures for surgical site infections.

We are taking care of sicker patients for longer, keeping them alive on vents far longer than they would have lived in the past. If a patient is on a vent for four weeks, that patient is likely to get pneumonia, even if the precautions are taken, and possibly develop C. *difficile* in spite of handwashing efforts and judicious use of antibiotics. These are facts of life, but hospitals can't just throw up their hands. They still need to take continuous action toward prevention and put resources into the program.

At the same time, we are faced with decisions regarding culturing patients on admission. If we do, will we isolate everyone who is colonized with MRSA or even VRE? And if positive, do we try to decolonize those patients? Will we be creating more resistance or opening the door to c. *difficile* if we begin treating everyone who is positive, even if they do not show any signs or symptoms of infection? None of these questions have been answered as yet, but the CDC multidrug-resistant organism guidelines address some of them. As this book went to press, the CDC was in the processing of releasing its new isolation guidelines. Link to them at *www.cdc.gov/ncidod/dhqp/gl_isolation_pt1.html.*

Partner with your risk manager and make certain he or she is aware of infections in the facility that could potentially lead to litigation issues. Make certain any infection that falls into the area of a sentinel event receives a root-cause analysis. Even if nothing more comes out of a case investigation than the paperwork, the fact that you looked at it works in your favor.

Staff education and public education are key components of your program. Fact sheets, like the one in Figure 7.1, for staff and the public are one way to continually educate.

Figure 7.1 — **CA-MRSA FACT SHEET**

FACT SHEET
Community Acquired MRSA

History

- Community-associated (CA) MRSA infections were first recognized in the 1980s.

- Persons with CA-MRSA infections are typically younger and healthier than persons with healthcare-associated MRSA.

- CA-MRSA bacteria are usually susceptible to more types of antibiotics than are healthcare-associated strains of MRSA.

Transmission

- Traditionally MRSA infections have been associated with hospitalization or other healthcare-associated risk factors, but in recent years physicians and other healthcare providers have observed an increasing number of people with MRSA infections who lack traditional healthcare-associated risk factors. These people appear to have community-associated infections.

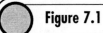

Figure 7.1

CA-MRSA FACT SHEET (CONT.)

Common Causes

• CA-MRSA infections can cause the same type of infections as other strains of staph. Studies conducted in Minnesota have found that CA-MRSA is more likely to cause skin and soft tissue infections and that healthcare-associated MRSA is more likely to be found in sputum or urine.

Signs and symptoms of infection
Most infections caused by *S. aureus* are skin and soft tissue infections such as abscesses or cellulitis.

Abscess

• Pocket of infection that forms at the site of injury.

• Usually filled with pus.

• Area surrounding the abscess is usually red, painful, and swollen and the skin surrounding the abscess can feel warm to the touch.

Cellulitis

• An infection of the underlying layers of the skin.

• Usually results from a scrape or cut in the skin which allows bacteria to enter, although no injury may be apparent.

• Cellulitis can occur anywhere in the body, but most often occurs on the legs or arms.

• Symptoms include redness, swelling, and pain at the site of infection.

S. aureus can also cause serious infections such as pneumonia (infection of the lungs) or bacteremia (bloodstream infection). Symptoms of these infections include: difficulty breathing, malaise, fever, or chills.

If you suspect you may have an infection with *S. aureus* contact your healthcare provider.

Duration of illness

• Some people can be colonized with *S. aureus* and never get an infection. For those people who do get an infection, the time from exposure to development of disease can be from days to years.

• Many common skin infections caused by *S. aureus* will heal without medical treatment. However, some skin infections will require incision and drainage of the infected site and some infections may require antibiotics.

Figure 7.1

CA-MRSA Fact Sheet (cont.)

- Most skin infections will heal within a few weeks, but more serious skin infections can take longer to heal if treatment is delayed or if ineffective treatment is given.

- More serious types of *S. aureus* infections (such as pneumonia or bloodstream infections) typically require hospitalization and treatment with intravenous antibiotics.

Complications

- There is a possibility for longer lasting or more severe infections with CA-MRSA if the initial antibiotic prescribed is not capable of killing the bacteria.

- Most skin infections resolve without treatment, however, some infections require incision and drainage or antibiotic treatment to cure the infection.

- Skin infections that are left untreated can develop into more serious life-threatening infections such as infections of the bone or blood.

- Some people experience repeated infections with *S. aureus*.

Unlike other strains of methicillin-resistant *Staphylococcus aureus*, community-acquired MRSA seems to spread rather easily, especially in families. Consequently, family members require some education about how to prevent transmission of the organism. First, the person who changes the wound dressing should dispose of old dressings in such a way that other family members won't be exposed. This person should also wash his or her hands meticulously after changing the dressing. The patient's towels, clothing, razors, dishes, and bed linens should not be used by other household members. The patient's laundry—including towels and bed linens—should be washed in hot water; sometimes bleach is recommended. It is not necessary, however, to perform nasal swabs on family members to determine if anyone is a carrier, as not all carriers develop the infection.

If, however, other household members do become ill with MRSA despite these precautions, it may be worth considering nasal colonization eradication techniques. One method is to apply mupirocin ointment to the nose twice daily. This provides only a short-term solution, but it may be sufficient to break the cycle of transmission. Chlorhexidine showers may also be helpful, and some infectious disease specialists recommend tub baths to which a half cup of bleach has been added.

Direct Care Staff: If you do direct patient care, remember to notify your immediate supervisor as well as the Employee Health Nurse if you have a draining lesion. If you are told that you have a strain of MRSA, you also need to notify your supervisor and Employee Health. They can determine whether or not you need to have your duties restricted in any way.

Construction

When construction goes on in your facility, continual diligence is essential. Involve your safety officer, construction foreman, and safety and environment of care committees. Safety during construction is not a one-person job and shouldn't fall to the ICP alone. The Joint Commission is looking to see that patient safety is a top concern as well as life safety measures.

We had construction going on both outside and inside our facility during our last Joint Commission survey. Surveyors noticed when a gate in the fence around a crane was left open. They noticed when workers tracked dust from inside a construction area into the rest of the hospital. Your IC delegate may have to round more than once a day to make certain walk off mats are used appropriately, air particulate matter is measured and negative pressure is used, air ducts sealed, and other measures are taken, especially during demolition. And remember, this can simply be revision or renovation of an area, as well as new construction.

Data presentation

Most facilities lean toward the data rich, information poor method of data collection. We produce all kinds of data on infections, resistant organism isolates, and hand hygiene, but are we able to present information with it? And how do we present it? Visuals, such as charts and graphs, are a great way to present information. In the book *Improving IC with Data* by Lorraine Duthe, BSN, MS, published by HCPro, the author demonstrates how to set up Excel spreadsheets to produce graphs.

In the graphs, it is essential to show the benchmark, average, and standard deviations above and below the average to see where you stand and whether the deviation is significant. Just because you know doesn't mean everyone else who sees a graph will know whether a spike is significant.

Arrows and text boxes to point out significant areas on graphs allow you to illustrate what the numbers mean. For example, on a graph documenting rates of ventilator-associated pneumonia (VAP), the rate might go from 4.5 infections per 1,000 ventilator days to 7.5 infections per 1,000 ventilator days, and yet you only had one infection each of those months. Someone will question that, so put in a box that says "ventilator days decreased this month." If an infection rate is 50%, but that reflects one out of two cases, that would be significant.

Why do we have to collect data?

- Compliance with The Joint Commission, the state health department, and other agencies
- Your own use
- For the patient
- Financial reasons

We've discussed data collection for agencies. Data collection for your own use as an ICP might include persuading administration to put money into IC-related improvements. Use central-line (CL) data to show how the use of antibiotic-impregnated dressings improved CL infection rates, saving the hospital money. When we introduced the impregnated dressings for central lines in our critical care unit, there was some skepticism since candidal blood stream infections (CBSI) rates were really low. With low rates, why make any changes? However, within a couple of months after making the change, our infection rates decreased by 50%. Even small changes can make a major impact.

You can collect data to improve patient satisfaction. If a patient ends up with an HAI, maybe a surgical site infection, he or she will have an increased length of stay, more discomfort, and in some cases, permanent disability. Also, because so much data is now publicly reported, patients will look at the data on sites like *www.hospitalcompare.com* and decide whether to come to your facility based on how you compare to other hospitals in your area. When you collect facility-specific data over time and compare it internally and externally, you have solid data you can use for decision-making. That gives you a good argument for directing financial resources in the most effective way for the IC program.

Effective program management

Modern hospital infection control (IC) programs first began in the 1950s in England, where their primary focus was to prevent and control healthcare-acquired staphylococcal outbreaks. In 1968, the American Hospital Association published *Infection Control in the Hospital*, a compendium of the first and only standards available for many years. At the same time, the Communicable Disease Center, later to be renamed the Centers for Disease Control and Prevention (CDC), began the first training courses specifically about IC and surveillance. In 1969, the Joint Commission for Accreditation of Hospitals—later to become The Joint Commission—first required hospitals to have organized IC committees (ICC) and isolation facilities.

In the 1970s, infection control underwent a growth spurt. By 1976, more than 50% of U.S. hospitals had a version of an IC program, including trained nurses to perform active surveillance. The CDC formed the Hospital Infections Branch and the Association for Practitioners in Infection Control was organized. By the close of the decade, the first CDC guidelines were written to answer frequently asked questions and establish consistent practice.

During the 1980s the cost value of IC programs was questioned. Then a combination of factors affecting healthcare impacted common IC practice. The first was the adoption of a fixed-price prospective payment system based on diagnostic-related groups (DRG), which resulted in wide-spread cost-containment initiatives to nonrevenue producing hospital services. IC was often included in that category. It was quickly discovered that a large number of DRGs did not allow for any complications or comorbidity. Most of the costs to treat nosocomial infections would not be reimbursed to hospitals. The fallout meant sicker patients were admitted into hospitals because less ill patients were treated on an outpatient basis or discharged earlier—a trend we continue to see in healthcare today, especially as surgeries like mastectomies and gall bladder removal become outpatient surgeries.

Another significant factor influencing IC was the advent of AIDS. HIV has taken an enormous toll in terms of loss of life and productivity. For IC professionals (ICP), HIV has been a challenge for education, risk reduction, and resource utilization.

In 1985, the *Study of the Efficacy of Nosocomial Infection Control* (SENIC) project was published, validating the cost-benefit of IC programs. Data collected in 1970 and 1976–1977 suggested that one-third of all nosocomial infections could be prevented if all the following were present:

- One ICP for every 250 beds
- An effective IC physician
- A program reporting infection rates back to the surgeon and those clinically involved with the infection
- An organized hospitalwide surveillance system

IC in the 1990s was influenced by the reform of the healthcare system when managed care networks became the preferred method for healthcare delivery. IC programs had to encompass not only hospitals but also long-term care facilities, home health/hospices, rehabilitation facilities, freestanding surgical centers, and physician office practices. A dramatic shift in patient care practices occurred, as greater than 65% of surgery cases were operated on in an outpatient setting. Issues that will continue to impact IC programs into the new millennium are a challenging combination of cost and clinical factors, including decreasing reimbursement, increasing cost to treat infections, and financial impact of implementing new government regulations.

ICP

From the beginning, the ICP has had to continually develop his or her practice as the field as developed. The Association for Professionals in Infection Control and Epidemiology (APIC) routinely surveys ICPs to determine the scope of practice for developing a national IC certification exam. Results suggest that regardless of the structure or hierarchy of the healthcare system, today's ICP needs knowledge of epidemiology statistics, patient care practices, occupational health, sterilization, disinfection, sanitation, infectious diseases, microbiology, education, and management.

The major responsibilities for ICPs to oversee include surveillance, specific environmental monitoring, continuous quality improvement, consultation, committee involvement, outbreak and isolation management, regulatory compliance, and education. To plan, coordinate, and succeed in fulfilling these responsibilities, many ICPs have to redefine their roles. More ICPs are becoming managers by creating multidisciplinary support teams to carry out many of the functions.

In addition to the ICP, healthcare systems should have an identified IC committee chair. This position is usually filled by a person who is a physician or who has a doctoral degree. The Joint Commission standards place an emphasis on documenting the specific epidemiologic and IC training of this individual. In large academic settings, a well-trained hospital epidemiologist can provide clinical and epidemiologic consultation.

The small community hospital often does not have an infectious disease physician at all. In these cases, the ICC chair will usually come from a specialty area such as pathology/laboratory, surgery, or medicine. In all areas, it is the ICP who must critically lead the IC program through daily activities.

Education

Education programs for employees and volunteers are one method to ensure competent IC practices. Educating the community, as well, is coming to the forefront as more emphasis is placed on prevention. You want visitors and family to adhere to IC principles like hand and respiratory hygiene. And educating staff is a unique challenge because employees represent a wide range of expertise and educational background. The ICP must become knowledgeable in adult education principles and use tools and techniques that will motivate and sustain behavioral change. Much has been written about the education of healthcare workers (HCW). Two side issues are how much education we should hand out and whether a knowledgeable public means more litigation.

Some of the tools used to successfully educate HCWs include newsletters, posters, and videos. Technological advances have also made video and telephone conferences opportunities for collaboration as well as teaching with few boundaries.

Whatever education methods you choose, IC programs must maintain training records of employees. The minimum training required are annual Occupational Safety and Health Administration bloodborne pathogen, tuberculosis prevention and control, and new employee orientation trainings.

ICPs should attend a basic IC-training course that is available through APIC, several university-based programs, or area APIC chapters. Other continuing education options are available through such professional organizations Society for Healthcare Epidemiology of America (SHEA), and APIC. Each organization holds annual educational conferences. Additionally, local APIC chapters offer education-al conferences. Locally, ICPs can participate in infectious disease or grand rounds at area hospitals. Taking courses on educating adults, computer technology, and epidemiology and statistics is also a good idea and may be available at local colleges.

Policies and procedures

ICPs must oversee the ongoing review and evaluation of written policies and procedures outlining prevention and control mechanisms in all patient care and service areas. Your policies and proce-dures should be based on recognized guidelines and applicable laws and regulations and should address the prevention of infection transmission among patients, employees, medical staff, contrac-tors, volunteers, visitors, and environmental issues. You should review/revise policies annually. Your IC manual must reflect what is actual practice in the institution because the organization is legally accountable for complying with its own policies. So although you don't have to reinvent the wheel, if you use a policy based on one from another facility, make certain it matches your own practice.

Regulatory compliance

Increasingly, IC programs have faced overwhelming demands from multiple regulatory authorities . The Joint Commission has redesigned its standards seeking outcome-oriented or performance improvement measurements. The Federal Drug Administration passed regulations to manage reprocessed single-use medical devices in its *Guidance on Enforcement Priorities for Single-Use Devices Reprocessed by Third Parties and Hospitals*. This document stipulates that reprocessed devices must meet the same requirements of newly manufactured devices. Therefore, hospitals and other third-party reprocessors who process these devices for reuse have to follow the same requirements as the initial manufacturer.

The CDC with the Hospital Infection Control Practices Advisory Committee has produced or revised several major guidelines. APIC has developed several guidelines covering topics including antisepsis and handwashing, disinfection and sterilization, endoscopy, and long-term care. In addition, each state has rules and laws for licensure, sanitation, and institutional kitchens. Each state has communi-cable disease rules to protect the general public health and medical waste laws. All of these guide-lines, standards, regulations, and laws must be interpreted and implemented for each healthcare organization—regardless of the size—to prevent citation, fines, litigation, and negative publicity.

Significant new trends in healthcare are occurring everyday, including medical procedures (e.g., gene therapy), technology (e.g., multipurpose IV catheters), and a shift from inpatient to outpatient care. Further changes in reimbursement and the push to reduce the cost of healthcare services with cuts in Medicaid/Medicare and managed care reimbursements mean even less money is available for healthcare. Survival of IC programs will depend on whether ICPs can efficiently demonstrate and communicate their value and provide competent and effective services. The Joint Commission standards have resulted in a dispersion of responsibility, but the ICP within the IC program will remain the facilitator for the broad scope of practice to prevent and control infections throughout the healthcare system.

Collaboration

Not only does a successful IC program require collaboration between the ICP, IC physician, hospital administration, clinical departments, and others, it requires broad collaboration—such as with the health department. But every bit as important is collaboration between ICPs. Both the local chapters of organizations such as APIC and national meetings will allow you to meet and greet other ICPs facing the same issues you do. When you meet with others who are struggling with IC and construction and core measures, you feel much less alone. As ICPs, we might begin to feel like a failure because our staff is the only group of HCWs in the country who fail to put on gloves to start an IV or draw a blood glucose. But this is wrong. There is a much bigger, universal problem that all ICPs fight every day.

Get all the e-mail addresses you can, join lists, keep in touch. If you want to begin something new at your own facility, other ICPs can tell you what they are doing in other area hospitals. If you are in close contact with other ICPs, you don't have to reinvent. They will let you borrow their ideas, or you could become a mentor yourself.

Tracers

When The Joint Commission comes, whether it's for your unannounced survey or the periodic review, you should have an IC tracer. You may see a tabletop tracer where the surveyor essentially interviews the entire ICC. Or you may actually see a patient tracer where you follow a patient from admission to discharge, through every unit the patient visited. In the tabletop tracer, Joint Commission surveyors will look at the involvement of each committee member and his or her ability to speak to actions taken, evaluations completed, and accomplishments by the committee.

When a patient is followed unit to unit, surveyors will examine communication between departments, watching how well the caregivers communicate with each other. For example, how will radiology be notified that a patient is in isolation before they walk in? If a patient is admitted to the med-surg unit from another facility through the emergency department (ED), will the information be transmitted that the patient was isolated for C. *diff*? The other facility might have told the ED, but will the ED remember to pass on that information? If the ED does not, will the nurses use critical thinking and notice the ED physician note saying the patient had "diarrhea, possibly infectious" and place the patient in isolation without a culture that specifies C. *difficile*?

When a practice tracer is done, pay particular attention to hand-hygiene compliance in general. With hand hygiene being so high profile and part of The Joint Commission's National Patient Safety Goals, you won't have too many chances to show compliance.

Resources

HICPAC: Healthcare IC Practices Advisory Committee
www.cdc.gov/ncidod/hip/hicpac/hicpac.htm
Morbidity and Mortality Weekly Report: http://www.cdc.gov/mmwr
OSHA: *www.osha.gov*

Hot list: Critical issues for infection control

CA-MRSA

Community-acquired MRSA is commonly seen in the ER, but may be admitted and pose a threat to hospitalized patients. Key indicators:

- Skin lesion
- Younger person, no hospital or antibiotic history
- Often presents to ER as an infected "bug bite" or "spider bite"
- May present in multiple sites
- Often returns same site or another
- Frequently seen in children and athletes due to close contact in school, on teams, sharing equipment
- If admitted, make certain contact isolation is in place
- Potential for severe invasive disease, including necrotizing pneumonia, necrotizing fasciitis, sever osteomyelitis, and a sepsis syndrome with increased mortality have been described in children and adults

MRSA

Patients colonized with MRSA often are more likely to develop symptomatic infections, with higher case fatality rates, according to the CDC's MDRO Guidelines, published in October 2006. The prevalence of MRSA has increased since first isolated in 1968. From the 1990s, when MRSA accounted for

20% to 25% of *Staphylococcus aureus* isolates from hospitalized patients to 2003, where 59.5% of S. *aureus* isolates in NNIS ICUs were MRSA.

- MDROs are carried from one person to another via the hands of healthcare professionals.
- Education that is facilitywide, unit-targeted, and informal educational interventions that encourage behavioral change
- Judicious use of antimicrobial agents
- Surveillance, including antibiograms
- Infection rates in specific populations, i.e., ICU, NICU
- Active surveillance cultures (ASC) to detect asymptomatic colonization is still being debated as an effective action.
- Standard and Contact Precautions most often used in combination, until patient is discharged, even with colonization
- Environmental cleaning that focuses on increased cleaning and disinfection of frequently-touched surfaces (e.g., bedrails, charts, bedside commodes, doorknobs)
- Decolonization has rarely been successful except for those who carry MRSA in their nares

TB

The U.S. rate of tuberculosis has been steadily declining; however, the heathcare programs that have helped lessen the spread of TB nationwide are losing steam. The rate of decline has not met the case-rate goal set for 2004. New TB guidelines from the CDC were released in 2005.

- All settings are required to perform a TB risk assessment annually
- All settings must evaluate their TB program annually
- Less TB testing may be required for some settings depending upon their risk assessment
- New recommendations for annual respiratory training, initial fit testing, and periodic testing
- Recommendation for TST rather than PPD

See the CDCs TB guidelines at *www.cdc.gov*.

Immunization

The Joint Commission in standard IC. Recommends immunization of all healthcare personnel, LIPs, and volunteers with influenza vaccine.

- Includes all staff, volunteers and licensed independent practitioners
- Vaccine must be offered to everyone who is eligible
- The program must be tracked for compliance and reassessed for effectiveness
- Percentages of vaccination are to be tracked

NPSG

The National Patient Safety Goal from The Joint Commission covers many of the hospital functions that involve patient safety. The one of most concern for ICPs is goal #7 regarding the prevention of healthcare-associated infections by:

- Compliance with the CDC's hand-hygiene guidelines
  - Which must be monitored in all settings
  - The results communicated to the settings
  - Actions taken to improve compliance
- Infections resulting in death and not related to admitting diagnoses are treated as sentinel events and a root-cause analysis is performed.

Core measures

This set of measures covers multiple diagnosis and recommends physician and staff compliance with certain actions designed to improve patient outcomes. The infection control measures revolve around Surgical Care Improvement Measures regarding infection prevention by compliance with prophylactic antibiotic recommendations.

The greatest impact on the ICP is the chart abstraction and data management required to publicly report the results in compliance with the reporting guidelines set out by CMS.

Pandemics

Pandemic planning, influx of infectious patients planning, and influenza planning all fall under the disaster management planning for a facility. We have fallen into the trap of multiple boutique plans for specific diseases like SARS, actions such as bioterrorism, and/or an influenza pandemic. My recommendation is to work with the safety officer to design a plan that deals with patient influx of any kind, including infectious patients due to an outbreak, bioterrorism, or a pandemic. Otherwise, staff has to deal with finding the right plan for the right disease or disaster.

Emerging and reemerging diseases/outbreaks

With emerging and reemerging diseases, the key issue is keeping informed, whether the issue is a new Pertussis outbreak or, the latest E. coli-0157 spinach contamination. Stay in constant communication with your local and state health departments for updates as well as monitoring the CDC sites.

Keep your staff informed in a timely manner. Even though they work in healthcare they look upon you as the expert and depend on you to keep them informed so they can protect themselves, their families, and their patients.

C. Difficile

C. *difficile* has become more prevalent with the continual use and misuse of antibiotics. Patients with a longer length of stay combined with multiple antibiotics often acquire C. *difficile*. However, some cases have been documented in relatively healthy individuals who have not received antibiotics, been hospitalized, or have an immune-compromised status.

- Contact precautions
- Environmental cleaning daily to include all horizontal and frequently touched surfaces
- Evaluation of antibiotics
- Wash hands with soap and water, do not use alcohol products alone

Device-related infections

VAP

Bundled, evidence based practices are often the best preventative measure for device related infections such as ventilator-associated pneumonia. Measures would include:

- Routine mouth care
- Elevated HOB 30-45 degrees
- Daily evaluations to see of they can be extubated
- Daily dedation vacation
- Deep vein thrombosis and peptic ulcer disease prophylaxis

CBSI

- Keep it sterile. Central line procedures require gull gowns and gloves when inserting, cleansing of skins with appropriate disinfectants, and full-sized drape. Hospital staff should wear face masks.
- Sterile material cart for CL dressing changes.
- Strict hand-hygiene compliance

Construction

Ec.8.30 requires a risk assessment before a project to identify patient hazards, determine how the project affects air quality, infections control, utilities, etc., and the use of controls to reduce risk to the patient population.

- Use sticky mats to remove dust from shoes to prevent dust tracking out of construction areas into patient areas
- Use negative pressure for the construction area to keep contaminants away from patients
- Barriers need to be made from impervious materials and sealed with duct tape
- Test soil for aspergillus and other contaminates before breaking ground on a project that will later be tied into the facility's HVAC system

For a rundown of the new AIA guidelines look at *www.ashe.org* in the "Education Quick Links" section.

CDC MDRO policy

On the following pages is the long-awaited guideline, *Management of Multidrug-Resistant Organisms in Healthcare Settings*, from the Centers for Disease Control and Prevention. For the full document, including list of authors, go to *http://www.cdc.gov/ncidod/dhqp/pdf/ar/mdroGuideline2006.pdf* (accessed January 16, 2007).

Management of Multidrug-Resistant Organisms In Healthcare Settings, 2006

Jane D. Siegel, MD; Emily Rhinehart, RN MPH CIC; Marguerite Jackson, PhD; Linda Chiarello, RN MS; the Healthcare Infection Control Practices Advisory Committee

Acknowledgement:
The authors and HICPAC gratefully acknowlege Dr. Larry Strausbaugh for his many contributions and valued guidance in the preparation of this guideline.

MDRO POLICY (CONT.)

I. Introduction

Multidrug-resistant organisms(MDROs), including methicillin-resistant *Staphylococcus aureus* (MRSA), vancomycin-resistant enterococci (VRE) and certain gram-negative bacilli (GNB) have important infection control implications that either have not been addressed or received only limited consideration in previous isolation guidelines. Increasing experience with these organisms is improving understanding of the routes of transmission and effective preventive measures. Although transmission of MDROs is most frequently documented in acute care facilities, all healthcare settings are affected by the emergence and transmission of antimicrobial-resistant microbes. The severity and extent of disease caused by these pathogens varies by the population(s) affected and by the institution(s) in which they are found. Institutions, in turn, vary widely in physical and functional characteristics, ranging from long-term care facilities (LTCF) to specialty units (e.g., intensive care units [ICU], burn units, neonatal ICUs [NICUs]) in tertiary care facilities. Because of this, the approaches to prevention and control of these pathogens need to be tailored to the specific needs of each population and individual institution. The prevention and control of MDROs is a national priority - one that requires that all healthcare facilities and agencies assume responsibility(1) (2). The following discussion and recommendations are provided to guide the implementation of strategies and practices to prevent the transmission of MRSA, VRE, and other MDROs. The administration of healthcare organizations and institutions should ensure that appropriate strategies are fully implemented, regularly evaluated for effectiveness, and adjusted such that there is a consistent decrease in the incidence of targeted MDROs. Successful prevention and control of MDROs requires administrative and scientific leadership and a financial and human resource commitment(3-5). Resources must be made available for infection prevention and control, including expert consultation, laboratory support, adherence monitoring, and data analysis. Infection prevention and control professionals have found that healthcare personnel (HCP) are more receptive and adherent to the recommended control measures when organizational leaders participate in efforts to reduce MDRO transmission(3).

Appendix B

II. Background

MDRO definition*. For* epidemiologic purposes, MDROs are defined as microorganisms, predominantly bacteria, that are resistant to one or more classes of antimicrobial agents (1). Although the names of certain MDROs describe resistance to only one agent (e.g., MRSA, VRE), these pathogens are frequently resistant to most available antimicrobial agents . These highly resistant organisms deserve special attention in healthcare facilities (2). In addition to MRSA and VRE, certain GNB, including those producing extended spectrum beta-lactamases (ESBLs) and others that are resistant to multiple classes of antimicrobial agents, are of particular concern.[1] In addition to *Escherichia coli* and *Klebsiella pneumoniae*, these include strains of *Acinetobacter baumannii* resistant to all antimicrobial agents, or all except imipenem,(6-12), and organisms such as *Stenotrophomonas maltophilia* (12-14), *Burkholderia cepacia (15, 16)*, and *Ralstonia pickettii(17)* that are intrinsically resistant to the broadest-spectrum antimicrobial agents. In some residential settings (e.g., LTCFs), it is important to control multidrug-resistant *S. pneumoniae* (MDRSP) that are resistant to penicillin and other broad-spectrum agents such as macrolides and fluroquinolones (18, 19). Strains of *S. aureus* that have intermediate susceptibility or are resistant to vancomycin (i.e., vancomycin-intermediate *S. aureus* [VISA], vancomycin-resistant *S. aureus* [VRSA]) (20-30) have affected specific populations, such as hemodialysis patients.

Clinical importance of MDROs*.* In most instances, MDRO infections have clinical manifestations that are similar to infections caused by susceptible pathogens. However, options for treating patients with these infections are often extremely limited. For example, until recently, only vancomycin provided effective therapy for potentially life-threatening MRSA infections and during the 1990's there were virtually no antimicrobial agents to treat infections caused by VRE. Although antimicrobials are now available for treatment of MRSA and VRE infections, resistance to each new agent has already emerged in clinical

---

1 Multidrug-resistant strains of *M. tuberculosis* are not addressed in this document because of the markedly different patterns of transmission and spread of the pathogen and the very different control interventions that are needed for prevention of *M. tuberculosis* infection. Current recommendations for prevention and control of tuberculosis can be found at: http://www.cdc.gov/mmwr/pdf/rr/rr5417.pdf

MDRO POLICY (CONT.)

isolates(31-37). Similarly, therapeutic options are limited for ESBL-producing isolates of gram-negative bacilli, strains of *A. baumannii* resistant to all antimicrobial agents except imipenem(8-11, 38) and intrinsically resistant *Stenotrophomonas* sp.(12-14, 39). These limitations may influence antibiotic usage patterns in ways that suppress normal flora and create a favorable environment for development of colonization when exposed to potential MDR pathogens (i.e., selective advantage)(40).

Increased lengths of stay, costs, and mortality also have been associated with MDROs (41-46). Two studies documented increased mortality, hospital lengths of stay, and hospital charges associated with multidrug-resistant gram-negative bacilli (MDR-GNBs), including an NICU outbreak of ESBL-producing *Klebsiella pneumoniae* (47) and the emergence of third-generation cephalosporin resistance in *Enterobacter* spp. in hospitalized adults (48). Vancomycin resistance has been reported to be an independent predictor of death from enterococcal bacteremia(44, 49-53). Furthermore, VRE was associated with increased mortality, length of hospital stay, admission to the ICU, surgical procedures, and costs when VRE patients were compared with a matched hospital population (54).

However, MRSA may behave differently from other MDROs. When patients with MRSA have been compared to patients with methicillin-susceptible *S. aureus* (MSSA), MRSA-colonized patients more frequently develop symptomatic infections(55, 56). Furthermore, higher case fatality rates have been observed for certain MRSA infections, including bacteremia(57-62), poststernotomy mediastinitis(63), and surgical site infections(64). These outcomes may be a result of delays in the administration of vancomycin, the relative decrease in the bactericidal activity of vancomycin(65), or persistent bacteremia associated with intrinsic characteristics of certain MRSA strains (66). Mortality may be increased further by *S. aureus* with reduced vancomycin susceptibility (VISA) (26, 67). Also some studies have reported an association between MRSA infections and increased length of stay, and healthcare costs(46, 61, 62), while others have not(64). Finally, some hospitals have observed an increase in the overall occurrence of staphylococcal infections following the introduction of MRSA into a hospital or special-care unit(68, 69).

III. Epidemiology of MDROs

Trends: Prevalence of MDROs varies temporally, geographically, and by healthcare setting(70, 71). For example, VRE emerged in the eastern United States in the early 1990s, but did not appear in the western United States until several years later, and MDRSP varies in prevalence by state(72). The type and level of care also influence the prevalence of MDROs. ICUs, especially those at tertiary care facilities, may have a higher prevalence of MDRO infections than do non-ICU settings (73, 74). Antimicrobial resistance rates are also strongly correlated with hospital size, tertiary-level care, and facility type (e.g., LTCF)(75, 76). The frequency of clinical infection caused by these pathogens is low in LTCFs(77, 78). Nonetheless, MDRO infections in LTCFs can cause serious disease and mortality, and colonized or infected LTCF residents may serve as reservoirs and vehicles for MDRO introduction into acute care facilities (78-88). Another example of population differences in prevalence of target MDROs is in the pediatric population. Point prevalence surveys conducted by the Pediatric Prevention Network (PPN) in eight U.S. PICUs and 7 U.S. NICUs in 2000 found $\leq$ 4% of patients were colonized with MRSA or VRE compared with 10-24% were colonized with ceftazidime- or aminoglycoside-resistant gram-negative bacilli; < 3% were colonized with ESBL-producing gram negative bacilli. Despite some evidence that MDRO burden is greatest in adult hospital patients, MDRO require similar control efforts in pediatric populations as well(89).

During the last several decades, the prevalence of MDROs in U.S. hospitals and medical centers has increased steadily(90, 91). MRSA was first isolated in the United States in 1968. By the early 1990s, MRSA accounted for 20%-25% of *Staphylococcus aureus* isolates from hospitalized patients(92). In 1999, MRSA accounted for >50% of *S. aureus* isolates from patients in ICUs in the National Nosocomial Infection Surveillance (NNIS) system; in 2003, 59.5% of *S. aureus* isolates in NNIS ICUs were MRSA (93). A similar rise in prevalence has occurred with VRE (94). From 1990 to 1997, the prevalence of VRE in enterococcal isolates from hospitalized patients increased from <1% to approximately 15% (95). VRE accounted for almost 25% of enterococcus isolates in NNIS ICUs in 1999 (94), and 28.5% in 2003 (93).

MDRO POLICY (CONT.)

GNB resistant to ESBLs, fluoroquinolones, carbapenems, and aminoglycosides also have increased in prevalence. For example, in 1997, the SENTRY Antimicrobial Surveillance Program found that among *K. pneumoniae* strains isolated in the United States, resistance rates to ceftazidime and other third-generation cephalosporins were 6.6%, 9.7%, 5.4%, and 3.6% for bloodstream, pneumonia, wound, and urinary tract infections, respectively (95) In 2003, 20.6% of all *K. pneumoniae* isolates from NNIS ICUs were resistant to these drugs ((93)). Similarly, between 1999 and 2003, *Pseudomonas aeruginosa* resistance to fluoroquinolone antibiotics increased from 23% to 29.5% in NNIS ICUs(74). Also, a 3-month survey of 15 Brooklyn hospitals in 1999 found that 53% of *A. baumannii* strains exhibited resistance to carbapenems and 24% of *P. aeruginosa* strains were resistant to imipenem (10). During 1994-2000, a national review of ICU patients in 43 states found that the overall susceptibility to ciprofloxacin decreased from 86% to 76% and was temporally associated with increased use of fluoroquinolones in the United States (96).

Lastly, an analysis of temporal trends of antimicrobial resistance in non-ICU patients in 23 U.S. hospitals during 1996-1997 and 1998-1999 (97) found significant increases in the prevalence of resistant isolates including MRSA, ciprofloxacin-resistant *P. aeruginosa*, and ciprofloxacin- or ofloxacin-resistant *E. coli*. Several factors may have contributed to these increases including: selective pressure exerted by exposure to antimicrobial agents, particularly fluoroquinolones, outside of the ICU and/or in the community(7, 96, 98); increasing rates of community-associated MRSA colonization and infection(99, 100); inadequate adherence to infection control practices; or a combination of these factors.

Important concepts in transmission. Once MDROs are introduced into a healthcare setting, transmission and persistence of the resistant strain is determined by the availability of vulnerable patients, selective pressure exerted by antimicrobial use, increased potential for transmission from larger numbers of colonized or infected patients ("colonization pressure")(101, 102); and the impact of implementation and adherence to prevention efforts. Patients vulnerable to colonization and infection include those with severe disease, especially those with compromised host defenses from underlying medical conditions; recent surgery; or indwelling medical devices (e.g., urinary catheters or endotracheal tubes(103, 104)). Hospitalized patients, especially ICU patients, tend to have more risk factors than non-hospitalized patients do, and have the highest infection rates. For example, the risk that an ICU patient will acquire VRE increases significantly once the proportion of ICU patients colonized with VRE exceeds 50%(101) or the number days of exposure to a VRE-patient exceeds 15 days(105). A similar effect of colonization pressure has been demonstrated for MRSA in a medical ICU(102). Increasing numbers of infections with MDROs also have been reported in non-ICU areas of hospitals(97).

There is ample epidemiologic evidence to suggest that MDROs are carried from one person to another via the hands of HCP(106-109). Hands are easily contaminated during the process of care-giving or from contact with environmental surfaces in close proximity to the patient(110-113). The latter is especially important when patients have diarrhea and the reservoir of the MDRO is the gastrointestinal tract(114-117). Without adherence to published recommendations for hand hygiene and glove use(111) HCP are more likely to transmit MDROs to patients. Thus, strategies to increase and monitor adherence are important components of MDRO control programs(106, 118).

Opportunities for transmission of MDROs beyond the acute care hospital results from patients receiving care at multiple healthcare facilities and moving between acute-care, ambulatory and/or chronic care, and LTC environments. System-wide surveillance at LDS Hospital in Salt Lake City, Utah, monitored patients identified as being infected or colonized with MRSA or VRE, and found that those patients subsequently received inpatient or outpatient care at as many as 62 different healthcare facilities in that system during a 5-year span(119).

Role of colonized HCP in MDRO transmission. Rarely, HCP may introduce an MDRO into a patient care unit(120-123). Occasionally, HCP can become persistently colonized with an MDRO, but these HCP have a limited role in transmission, unless other factors are present. Additional factors that can facilitate transmission, include chronic sinusitis(120), upper respiratory infection(123), and dermatitis(124).

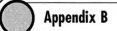 **Appendix B**

MDRO POLICY (CONT.)

Implications of community-associated MRSA (CA-MRSA). The emergence of new epidemic strains of MRSA in the community, among patients without established MRSA risk factors, may present new challenges to MRSA control in healthcare settings(125-128). Historically, genetic analyses of MRSA isolated from patients in hospitals worldwide revealed that a relatively small number of MRSA strains have unique qualities that facilitate their transmission from patient to patient within healthcare facilities over wide geographic areas, explaining the dramatic increases in HAIs caused by MRSA in the 1980s and early 1990s(129). To date, most MRSA strains isolated from patients with CA-MRSA infections have been microbiologically distinct from those endemic in healthcare settings, suggesting that some of these strains may have arisin *de novo* in the community via acquisition of methicillin resistance genes by established methicillin-susceptible *S. aureus* (MSSA) strains(130-132). Two pulsed-field types, termed USA300 and USA400 according to a typing scheme established at CDC, have accounted for the majority of CA-MRSA infections characterized in the United States, whereas pulsed-field types USA100 and USA200 are the predominant genotypes endemic in healthcare settings(133).

USA300 and USA400 genotypes almost always carry type IV of the staphylococcal chromosomal cassette (SCC) *mec*, the mobile genetic element that carries the *mec*A methicillin-resistance gene (133, 134). This genetic cassette is smaller than types I through III, the types typically found in healthcare associated MRSA strains, and is hypothesized to be more easily transferable between *S. aureus* strains.

CA-MRSA infection presents most commonly as relatively minor skin and soft tissue infections, but severe invasive disease, including necrotizing pneumonia, necrotizing fasciitis, severe osteomyelitis, and a sepsis syndrome with increased mortality have also been described in children and adults(134-136).

Transmission within hospitals of MRSA strains first described in the community (e.g. USA300 and USA400) are being reported with increasing frequency(137-140). Changing resistance patterns of MRSA in ICUs in the NNIS system from 1992 to 2003 provide additional evidence that the new epidemic MRSA strains are becoming established healthcare-associated as well as community pathogens(90). Infections with these strains have most commonly presented as skin disease in community settings. However, intrinsic virulence characteristics of the organisms can result in clinical manifestations similar to or potentially more severe than traditional healthcare-associated MRSA infections among hospitalized patients. The prevalence of MRSA colonization and infection in the surrounding community may therefore affect the selection of strategies for MRSA control in healthcare settings.

IV. MDRO Prevention and Control

Prevention of Infections. Preventing infections will reduce the burden of MDROs in healthcare settings. Prevention of antimicrobial resistance depends on appropriate clinical practices that should be incorporated into all routine patient care. These include optimal management of vascular and urinary catheters, prevention of lower respiratory tract infection in intubated patients, accurate diagnosis of infectious etiologies, and judicious antimicrobial selection and utilization. Guidance for these preventive practices include the Campaign to Reduce Antimicrobial Resistance in Healthcare Settings (www.cdc.gov/drugresistance/healthcare/default.htm), a multifaceted, evidence-based approach with four parallel strategies: infection prevention; accurate and prompt diagnosis and treatment; prudent use of antimicrobials; and prevention of transmission. Campaign materials are available for acute care hospitals, surgical settings, dialysis units, LTCFs and pediatric acute care units.

To reduce rates of central-venous-line associated bloodstream infections(CVL-BSIs) and ventilator-associated pneumonia (VAP), a group of bundled evidence-based clinical practices have been implemented in many U.S. healthcare facilities(118, 141-144). One report demonstrated a sustained effect on the reduction in CVL-BSI rates with this approach(145). Although the specific effect on MDRO infection and colonization rates have not been reported, it is logical that decreasing these and other healthcare-associated infections will in turn reduce antimicrobial use and decrease opportunities for emergence and transmission of MDROs.

MDRO POLICY (CONT.)

Prevention and Control of MDRO transmission

Overview of the MDRO control literature. Successful control of MDROs has been documented in the United States and abroad using a variety of combined interventions. These include improvements in hand hygiene, use of Contact Precautions until patients are culture-negative for a target MDRO, active surveillance cultures (ASC), education, enhanced environmental cleaning, and improvements in communication about patients with MDROs within and between healthcare facilities.

Representative studies include:

- Reduced rates of MRSA transmission in The Netherlands, Belgium, Denmark, and other Scandinavian countries after the implementation of aggressive and sustained infection control interventions (i.e., ASC; preemptive use of Contact Precautions upon admission until proven culture negative; and, in some instances, closure of units to new admissions). MRSA generally accounts for a very small proportion of *S. aureus* clinical isolates in these countries(146-150).

- Reduced rates of VRE transmission in healthcare facilities in the three-state Siouxland region (Iowa, Nebraska, and South Dakota) following formation of a coalition and development of an effective region-wide infection control intervention that included ASC and isolation of infected patients. The overall prevalence rate of VRE in the 30 participating facilities decreased from 2.2% in 1997 to 0.5% in 1999(151).

- Eradication of endemic MRSA infections from two NICUs. The first NICU included implementation of ASC, Contact Precautions, use of triple dye on the umbilical cord, and systems changes to improve surveillance and adherence to recommended practices and to reduce overcrowding(152). The second NICU used ASC and Contact Precautions; surgical masks were included in the barriers used for Contact Precautions(153).

- Control of an outbreak and eventual eradication of VRE from a burn unit over a 13-month period with implementation of aggressive culturing, environmental cleaning, and barrier isolation(154).

- Control of an outbreak of VRE in a NICU over a 3-year period with implementation of ASC, other infection control measures such as use of a waterless hand disinfectant, and mandatory in-service education(155).

- Eradication of MDR-strains of *A. baumannii* from a burn unit over a 16-month period with implementation of strategies to improve adherence to hand hygiene, isolation, environmental cleaning, and temporary unit closure(38).

- In addition, more than 100 reports published during 1982-2005 support the efficacy of combinations of various control interventions to reduce the burden of MRSA, VRE, and MDR-GNBs (Tables 1 and 2). Case-rate reduction or pathogen eradication was reported in a majority of studies.

- VRE was eradicated in seven special-care units(154, 156-160), two hospitals(161, 162), and one LTCF(163).

- MRSA was eradicated from nine special-care units(89, 152, 153, 164-169), two hospitals(170), one LTCF(167), and one Finnish district(171). Furthermore, four MRSA reports described continuing success in sustaining low endemic MDRO rates for over 5 years(68, 166, 172, 173).

- An MDR-GNB was eradicated from 13 special-care units(8, 9, 38, 174-180) and two hospitals (11, 181).

These success stories testify to the importance of having dedicated and knowledgeable teams of healthcare professionals who are willing to persist for years, if necessary, to control MDROs. Eradication and control of MDROs, such as those reported, frequently required periodic reassessment and the addition of new and more stringent interventions over time (tiered strategy). For example, interventions were added in a stepwise fashion during a 3-year effort that eventually eradicated MRSA from an NICU(152). A series of interventions was adopted throughout the course of a year to eradicate VRE from a burn unit(154). Similarly, eradication of carbapenem-resistant strains of *A. baumannii* from a hospital required multiple and progressively more intense interventions over several years(11).

Nearly all studies reporting successful MDRO control employed a median of 7 to 8 different interventions concurrently or sequentially (Table 1). These figures may underestimate the actual number of control measures used, because authors of these reports may have considered their earliest efforts routine (e.g., added emphasis on handwashing), and did not include them as interventions, and some "single measures" are, in fact, a complex

MDRO POLICY (CONT.)

combination of several interventions. The use of multiple concurrent control measures in these reports underscores the need for a comprehensive approach for controlling MDROs.

Several factors affect the ability to generalize the results of the various studies reviewed, including differences in definition, study design, endpoints and variables measured, and period of follow-up. Two-thirds of the reports cited in Tables 1 and 2 involved perceived outbreaks, and one-third described efforts to reduce endemic transmission. Few reports described preemptive efforts or prospective studies to control MDROs before they had reached high levels within a unit or facility.

With these and other factors, it has not been possible to determine the effectiveness of individual interventions, or a specific combination of interventions, that would be appropriate for all healthcare facilities to implement in order to control their target MDROs. Randomized controlled trials are necessary to acquire this level of evidence. An NIH-sponsored, randomized controlled trial on the prevention of MRSA and VRE transmission in adult ICUs is ongoing and may provide further insight into optimal control measures (http://clinicaltrials.gov/ct/show/NCT00100386?order=1). This trial compares the use of education (to improve adherence to hand hygiene) and Standard Precautions to the use of ASC and Contact Precautions.

Control Interventions. The various types of interventions used to control or eradicate MDROs may be grouped into seven categories. These include administrative support, judicious use of antimicrobials, surveillance (routine and enhanced), Standard and Contact Precautions, environmental measures, education and decolonization. These interventions provide the basis for the recommendations for control of MDROs in healthcare settings that follow this review and as summarized in Table 3. In the studies reviewed, these interventions were applied in various combinations and degrees of intensity, with differences in outcome.

   1. *Administrative support.* In several reports, administrative support and involvement were important for the successful control of the target MDRO(3, 152, 182-185), and authorities in infection control have strongly recommended such support(2, 106, 107,

186). There are several examples of MDRO control interventions that require administrative commitment of fiscal and human resources. One is the use of ASC(8, 38, 68, 107, 114, 151, 152, 167, 168, 183, 184, 187-192). Other interventions that require administrative support include: 1) implementing system changes to ensure prompt and effective communications e.g., computer alerts to identify patients previously known to be colonized/infected with MDROs(184, 189, 193, 194); 2), providing the necessary number and appropriate placement of hand washing sinks and alcohol-containing hand rub dispensers in the facility(106, 195); 3) maintaining staffing levels appropriate to the intensity of care required(152, 196-202); and 4) enforcing adherence to recommended infection control practices (e.g., hand hygiene, Standard and Contact Precautions) for MDRO control. Other measures that have been associated with a positive impact on prevention efforts, that require administrative support, are direct observation with feedback to HCP on adherence to recommended precautions and keeping HCP informed about changes in transmission rates(3, 152, 182, 203-205). A "How-to guide" for implementing change in ICUs, including analysis of structure, process, and outcomes when designing interventions, can assist in identification of needed administrative interventions(195). Lastly, participation in existing, or the creation of new, city-wide, state-wide, regional or national coalitions, to combat emerging or growing MDRO problems is an effective strategy that requires administrative support(146, 151, 167, 188, 206, 207).

2. *Education.* Facility-wide, unit-targeted, and informal, educational interventions were included in several successful studies(3, 189, 193, 208-211). The focus of the interventions was to encourage a behavior change through improved understanding of the problem MDRO that the facility was trying to control. Whether the desired change involved hand hygiene, antimicrobial prescribing patterns, or other outcomes, enhancing understanding and creating a culture that supported and promoted the desired behavior, were viewed as essential to the success of the intervention. Educational campaigns to enhance adherence to hand hygiene practices in conjunction with other control measures have been associated temporally with decreases in MDRO transmission in various healthcare settings(3, 106, 163).

MDRO POLICY (CONT.)

3. *Judicious use of antimicrobial agents.* While a comprehensive review of antimicrobial stewardship is beyond the scope of this guideline, recommendations for control of MDROs must include attention to judicious antimicrobial use. A temporal association between formulary changes and decreased occurrence of a target MDRO was found in several studies, especially in those that focused on MDR-GNBs(98, 177, 209, 212-218). Occurrence of C. difficile-associated disease has also been associated with changes in antimicrobial use(219). Although some MRSA and VRE control efforts have attempted to limit antimicrobial use, the relative importance of this measure for controlling these MDROs remains unclear(193, 220). Limiting antimicrobial use alone may fail to control resistance due to a combination of factors; including 1) the relative effect of antimicrobials on providing initial selective pressure, compared to perpetuating resistance once it has emerged; 2) inadequate limits on usage; or 3) insufficient time to observe the impact of this intervention. With the intent of addressing #2 and #3 above in the study design, one study demonstrated a decrease in the prevalence of VRE associated with a formulary switch from ticarcillin-clavulanate to piperacillin-tazobactam(221).

The CDC Campaign to Prevent Antimicrobial Resistance that was launched in 2002 provides evidence-based principles for judicious use of antimicrobials and tools for implementation(222) www.cdc.gov/drugresistance/healthcare. This effort targets all healthcare settings and focuses on effective antimicrobial treatment of infections, use of narrow spectrum agents, treatment of infections and not contaminants, avoiding excessive duration of therapy, and restricting use of broad-spectrum or more potent antimicrobials to treatment of serious infections when the pathogen is not known or when other effective agents are unavailable. Achieving these objectives would likely diminish the selective pressure that favors proliferation of MDROs. Strategies for influencing antimicrobial prescribing patterns within healthcare facilities include education; formulary restriction; prior-approval programs, including pre-approved indications; automatic stop orders; academic interventions to counteract pharmaceutical influences on prescribing patterns; antimicrobial cycling(223-226);

computer-assisted management programs(227-229); and active efforts to remove redundant antimicrobial combinations(230). A systematic review of controlled studies identified several successful practices. These include social marketing (i.e. consumer education), practice guidelines, authorization systems, formulary restriction, mandatory consultation, and peer review and feedback. It further suggested that online systems that provide clinical information, structured order entry, and decision support are promising strategies(231). These changes are best accomplished through an organizational, multidisciplinary, antimicrobial management program(232).

4. *MDRO surveillance.* Surveillance is a critically important component of any MDRO control program, allowing detection of newly emerging pathogens, monitoring epidemiologic trends, and measuring the effectiveness of interventions. Multiple MDRO surveillance strategies have been employed, ranging from surveillance of clinical microbiology laboratory results obtained as part of routine clinical care, to use of ASC to detect asymptomatic colonization.

Surveillance for MDROs isolated from routine clinical cultures.
Antibiograms. The simplest form of MDRO surveillance is monitoring of clinical microbiology isolates resulting from tests ordered as part of routine clinical care. This method is particularly useful to detect emergence of new MDROs not previously detected, either within an individual healthcare facility or community-wide. In addition, this information can be used to prepare facility- or unit-specific summary antimicrobial susceptibility reports that describe pathogen-specific prevalence of resistance among clinical isolates. Such reports may be useful to monitor for changes in known resistance patterns that might signal emergence or transmission of MDROs, and also to provide clinicians with information to guide antimicrobial prescribing practices(233-235).

MDRO Incidence Based on Clinical Culture Results. Some investigators have used clinical microbiology results to calculate measures of incidence of MDRO isolates in specific populations or patient care locations (e.g. new MDRO

MDRO POLICY (CONT.)

isolates/1,000 patient days, new MDRO isolates per month)(205, 236, 237). Such measures may be useful for monitoring MDRO trends and assessing the impact of prevention programs, although they have limitations. Because they are based solely on positive culture results without accompanying clinical information, they do not distinguish colonization from infection, and may not fully demonstrate the burden of MDRO-associated disease. Furthermore, these measures do not precisely measure acquisition of MDRO colonization in a given populaton or location. Isolating an MDRO from a clinical culture obtained from a patient several days after admission to a given unit or facility does not establish that the patient acquired colonization in that unit. On the other hand, patients who acquire MDRO colonization may remain undetected by clinical cultures(107). Despite these limitations, incidence measures based on clinical culture results may be highly correlated with actual MDRO transmission rates derived from information using ASC, as demonstrated in a recent multicenter study(237). These results suggest that incidence measures based on clinical cultures alone might be useful surrogates for monitoring changes in MDRO transmission rates.

MDRO Infection Rates. Clinical cultures can also be used to identify targeted MDRO infections in certain patient populations or units(238, 239). This strategy requires investigation of clinical circumstances surrounding a positive culture to distinguish colonization from infection, but it can be particularly helpful in defining the clinical impact of MDROs within a facility.

Molecular typing of MDRO isolates. Many investigators have used molecular typing of selected isolates to confirm clonal transmission to enhance understanding of MDRO transmission and the effect of interventions within their facility(38, 68, 89, 92, 138, 152, 190, 193, 236, 240).

Surveillance for MDROs by Detecting Asymptomatic Colonization
Another form of MDRO surveillance is the use of active surveillance cultures (ASC) to identify patients who are colonized with a targeted MDRO(38, 107, 241). This

approach is based upon the observation that, for some MDROs, detection of colonization may be delayed or missed completely if culture results obtained in the course of routine clinical care are the primary means of identifying colonized patients(8, 38, 107, 114, 151, 153, 167, 168, 183, 184, 187, 189, 191-193, 242-244). Several authors report having used ASC when new pathogens emerge in order to define the epidemiology of the particular agent(22, 23, 107, 190). In addition, the authors of several reports have concluded that ASC, in combination with use of Contact Precautions for colonized patients, contributed directly to the decline or eradication of the target MDRO(38, 68, 107, 151, 153, 184, 217, 242). However, not all studies have reached the same conclusion. Poor control of MRSA despite use of ASC has been described(245). A recent study failed to identify cross-transmission of MRSA or MSSA in a MICU during a 10 week period when ASC were obtained, despite the fact that culture results were not reported to the staff(246). The investigators suggest that the degree of cohorting and adherence to Standard Precautions might have been the important determinants of transmission prevention, rather than the use of ASC and Contact Precautions for MRSA-colonized patients. The authors of a systematic review of the literature on the use of isolation measures to control healthcare-associated MRSA concluded that there is evidence that concerted efforts that include ASC and isolation can reduce MRSA even in endemic settings. However, the authors also noted that methodological weaknesses and inadequate reporting in published research make it difficult to rule out plausible alternative explanations for reductions in MRSA acquisition associated with these interventions, and therefore concluded that the precise contribution of active surveillance and isolation alone is difficult to assess(247).

Mathematical modeling studies have been used to estimate the impact of ASC use in control of MDROs. One such study evaluating interventions to decrease VRE transmission indicated that use of ASC (versus no cultures) could potentially decrease transmission 39% and that with pre-emptive isolation plus ASC, transmission could be decreased 65%(248). Another mathematical model examining the use of ASC and isolation for control of MRSA predicted that isolating colonized or infected patients on the basis of clinical culture results is unlikely to be successful at controlling MRSA, whereas use of active surveillance and isolation can lead to successful control, even in settings where MRSA is highly endemic.(249) There is less literature on the use of ASC in controlling MDR-GNBs. Active surveillance cultures have been used as part of efforts to successful control of MDR-GNBs in outbreak settings. The experience with ASC as part of successful control efforts in endemic settings is mixed. One study reported successful reduction of extended-spectrum beta-lactamase –producing Enterobacteriaceae over a six year period using a multifaceted control program that included use of ASC(245). Other reports suggest that use of ASC is not necessary to control endemic MDR-GNBs.(250, 251).

More research is needed to determine the circumstances under which ASC are most beneficial(252), but their use should be considered in some settings, especially if other control measures have been ineffective. When use of ASC is incorporated into MDRO prevention programs, the following should be considered:

- The decision to use ASC as part of an infection prevention and control program requires additional support for successful implementation, including: 1) personnel to obtain the appropriate cultures, 2) microbiology laboratory personnel to process the cultures, 3) mechanism for communicating results to caregivers, 4) concurrent decisions about use of additional isolation measures triggered by a positive culture (e.g. Contact Precautions) and 5) mechanism for assuring adherence to the additional isolation measures.
- The populations targeted for ASC are not well defined and vary among published reports. Some investigators have chosen to target specific patient populations considered at high risk for MDRO colonization based on factors such as location (e.g. ICU with high MDRO rates), antibiotic exposure history, presence of underlying diseases, prolonged duration of stay, exposure to other MDRO-colonized patients, patients transferred from other facilities known to have a high prevalence of MDRO carriage, or having a history of recent hospital or nursing home stays(107, 151, 253). A more commonly employed strategy involves obtaining surveillance cultures from all patients admitted to units experiencing

high rates of colonization/infection with the MDROs of interest, unless they are already known to be MDRO carriers(153, 184, 242, 254). In an effort to better define target populations for active surveillance, investigators have attempted to create prediction rules to identify subpopulations of patients at high risk for colonization on hospital admission(255, 256). Decisions about which populations should be targeted for active surveillance should be made in the context of local determinations of the incidence and prevalence of MDRO colonization within the intervention facility as well as other facilities with whom patients are frequently exchanged(257).

- Optimal timing and interval of ASC are not well defined. In many reports, cultures were obtained at the time of admission to the hospital or intervention unit or at the time of transfer to or from designated units (e.g., ICU)(107). In addition, some hospitals have chosen to obtain cultures on a periodic basis [e.g., weekly(8, 153, 159) to detect silent transmission. Others have based follow-up cultures on the presence of certain risk factors for MDRO colonization, such as antibiotic exposure, exposure to other MDRO colonized patients, or prolonged duration of stay in a high risk unit(253).

- Methods for obtaining ASC must be carefully considered, and may vary depending upon the MDRO of interest.
    - MRSA: Studies suggest that cultures of the nares identify most patients with MRSA and perirectal and wound cultures can identify additional carriers(152, 258-261).
    - VRE: Stool, rectal, or perirectal swabs are generally considered a sensitive method for detection of VRE. While one study suggested that rectal swabs may identify only 60% of individuals harboring VRE, and may be affected by VRE stool density(262), this observation has not been reported elsewhere in the literature.
    - MDR-GNBs: Several methods for detection of MDR-GNBs have been employed, including use of peri-rectal or rectal swabs alone or in combination with oro-pharyngeal, endotracheal, inguinal, or wound cultures. The absence of standardized screening media for many gram-

negative bacilli can make the process of isolating a specific MDR-GNB a relatively labor-intensive process(38, 190, 241, 250).

  o Rapid detection methods: Using conventional culture methods for active surveillance can result in a delay of 2-3 days before results are available. If the infection control precautions (e.g., Contact Precautions) are withheld until the results are available, the desired infection control measures could be delayed. If empiric precautions are used pending negative surveillance culture results, precautions may be unnecessarily implemented for many, if not most, patients. For this reason, investigators have sought methods for decreasing the time necessary to obtain a result from ASC. Commercially available media containing chromogenic enzyme substrates (CHROMagar MRSA(263, 264) has been shown to have high sensitivity and specificity for identification of MRSA and facilitate detection of MRSA colonies in screening cultures as early as 16 hours after inoculation. In addition, real-time PCR-based tests for rapid detection of MRSA directly from culture swabs (< 1-2 hours) are now commercially available(265-267), as well as PCR-based tests for detection of vanA and van B genes from rectal swabs(268). The impact of rapid testing on the effectiveness of active surveillance as a prevention strategy, however, has not been fully determined. Rapid identification of MRSA in one study was associated with a significant reduction in MRSA infections acquired in the medical ICU, but not the surgical ICU(265). A mathematical model characterizing MRSA transmission dynamics predicted that, in comparison to conventional culture methods, the use of rapid detection tests may decrease isolation needs in settings of low-endemicity and result in more rapid reduction in prevalence in highly-endemic settings(249).

• Some MDRO control reports described surveillance cultures of healthcare personnel during outbreaks, but colonized or infected healthcare personnel are rarely the source of ongoing transmission, and this strategy should be reserved for settings in which specific healthcare personnel have been epidemiologically implicated in the transmission of MDROs(38, 92, 152-154, 188).

5. ***Infection Control Precautions.*** Since 1996 CDC has recommended the use of Standard and Contact Precautions for MDROs "judged by an infection control program…to be of special clinical and epidemiologic significance." This recommendation was based on general consensus and was not necessarily evidence-based. No studies have directly compared the efficacy of Standard Precautions alone versus Standard Precautions and Contact Precautions, with or without ASC, for control of MDROs. Some reports mention the use of one or both sets of precautions as part of successful MDRO control efforts; however, the precautions were not the primary focus of the study intervention(164, 190, 205, 269-271). The NIH-sponsored study mentioned earlier (Section: *Overview of the MDRO control literature*) may provide some answers, http://clinicaltrials.gov/ct/show/NCT00100386?order=1).

Standard Precautions have an essential role in preventing MDRO transmission, even in facilities that use Contact Precautions for patients with an identified MDRO. Colonization with MDROs is frequently undetected; even surveillance cultures may fail to identify colonized persons due to lack of sensitivity, laboratory deficiencies, or intermittent colonization due to antimicrobial therapy(262). Therefore, Standard Precautions must be used in order to prevent transmission from potentially colonized patients. Hand hygiene is an important component of Standard Precautions. The authors of the *Guideline for Hand Hygiene in Healthcare Settings(106)* cited nine studies that demonstrated a temporal relationship between improved adherence to recommended hand hygiene practices and control of MDROs. It is noteworthy that in one report the frequency of hand hygiene did not improve with use of Contact Precautions but did improve when gloves were used (per Standard Precautions) for contact with MDRO patients(272).

MDRO control efforts frequently involved changes in isolation practices, especially during outbreaks. In the majority of reports, Contact Precautions were implemented for all patients found to be colonized or infected with the target MDRO (See Table 2).

MDRO POLICY (CONT.)

Some facilities also preemptively used Contact Precautions, in conjunction with ASC, for all new admissions or for all patients admitted to a specific unit, until a negative screening culture for the target MDRO was reported(30, 184, 273).

Contact Precautions are intended to prevent transmission of infectious agents, including epidemiologically important microorganisms, which are transmitted by direct or indirect contact with the patient or the patient's environment. A single-patient room is preferred for patients who require Contact Precautions. When a single-patient room is not available, consultation with infection control is necessary to assess the various risks associated with other patient placement options (e.g., cohorting, keeping the patient with an existing roommate). HCP caring for patients on Contact Precautions should wear a gown and gloves for all interactions that may involve contact with the patient or potentially contaminated areas in the patient's environment. Donning gown and gloves upon room entry and discarding before exiting the patient room is done to contain pathogens, especially those that have been implicated in transmission through environmental contamination (e.g., VRE, *C. difficile,* noroviruses and other intestinal tract agents; RSV)(109, 111, 274-277).

Cohorting and other MDRO control strategies. In several reports, cohorting of patients(152, 153, 167, 183, 184, 188, 189, 217, 242), cohorting of staff(184, 217, 242, 278), use of designated beds or units(183, 184), and even unit closure(38, 146, 159, 161, 279, 280) were necessary to control transmission. Some authors indicated that implementation of the latter two strategies were the turning points in their control efforts; however, these measures usually followed many other actions to prevent transmission. In one, two-center study, moving MRSA-positive patients into single rooms or cohorting these patients in designated bays failed to reduce transmission in ICUs. However, in this study adherence to recommendations for hand hygiene between patient contacts was only 21%(281). Other published studies, including one commissioned by the American Institute of Architects and the Facility Guidelines Institute (www.aia.org/aah_gd_hospcons), have documented a beneficial relationship between private rooms and reduction in risk of acquiring MDROs(282). Additional studies are needed to define the specific contribution of using single-patient rooms and/or cohorting on preventing transmission of MDROs.

Duration of Contact Precautions. The necessary duration of Contact Precautions for patients treated for infection with an MDRO, but who may continue to be colonized with the organism at one or more body sites, remains an unresolved issue. Patients may remain colonized with MDROs for prolonged periods; shedding of these organisms may be intermittent, and surveillance cultures may fail to detect their presence(84, 250, 283). The 1995 HICPAC guideline for preventing the transmission of VRE suggested three negative stool/perianal cultures obtained at weekly intervals as a criterion for discontinuation of Contact Precautions(274). One study found these criteria generally reliable(284). However, this and other studies have noted a recurrence of VRE positive cultures in persons who subsequently receive antimicrobial therapy and persistent or intermittent carriage of VRE for more than 1 year has been reported(284-286). Similarly, colonization with MRSA can be prolonged(287, 288). Studies demonstrating initial clearance of MRSA following decolonization therapy have reported a high frequency of subsequent carriage(289, 290). There is a paucity of information in the literature on when to discontinue Contact Precautions for patients colonized with a MDR-GNB, possibly because infection and colonization with these MDROs are often associated with outbreaks. Despite the uncertainty about when to discontinue Contact Precautions, the studies offer some guidance. In the context of an outbreak, prudence would dictate that Contact Precautions be used indefinitely for all previously infected and known colonized patients. Likewise, if ASC are used to detect and isolate patients colonized with MRSA or VRE, and there is no decolonization of these patients, it is logical to assume that Contact Precautions would be used for the duration of stay in the setting where they were first implemented. In general, it seems reasonable to discontinue Contact Precautions when three or more surveillance cultures for the target MDRO are repeatedly negative over the course of a week or two in a patient who has not received antimicrobial therapy for several weeks, especially in the absence of a draining wound, profuse respiratory secretions, or evidence implicating the specific patient in ongoing transmission of the MDRO within the facility.

Barriers used for contact with patients infected or colonized with MDROs.
Three studies evaluated the use of gloves with or without gowns for all patient contacts to prevent VRE acquisition in ICU settings(30, 105, 273). Two of the studies showed that use of both gloves and gowns reduced VRE transmission(30, 105) while the third showed no difference in transmission based on the barriers used(273). One study in a LTCF compared the use of gloves only, with gloves plus contact isolation, for patients with four MDROs, including VRE and MRSA, and found no difference(86). However, patients on contact isolation were more likely to acquire MDR-*K. pneumoniae* strains that were prevalent in the facility; reasons for this were not specifically known. In addition to differences in outcome, differing methodologies make comparisons difficult. Specifically, HCP adherence to the recommended protocol, the influence of added precautions on the number of HCP-patient interactions, and colonization pressure were not consistently assessed.

Impact of Contact Precautions on patient care and well-being. There are limited data regarding the impact of Contact Precautions on patients. Two studies found that HCP, including attending physicians, were half as likely to enter the rooms of(291), or examine(292), patients on Contact Precautions. Other investigators have reported similar observations on surgical wards(293). Two studies reported that patients in private rooms and on barrier precautions for an MDRO had increased anxiety and depression scores(294, 295). Another study found that patients placed on Contact Precautions for MRSA had significantly more preventable adverse events, expressed greater dissatisfaction with their treatment, and had less documented care than control patients who were not in isolation(296). Therefore, when patients are placed on Contact Precautions, efforts must be made by the healthcare team to counteract these potential adverse effects.

6. ***Environmental measures.*** The potential role of environmental reservoirs, such as surfaces and medical equipment, in the transmission of VRE and other MDROs has been the subject of several reports(109-111, 297, 298). While environmental cultures are not routinely recommended(299), environmental cultures were used in several studies to document contamination, and led to interventions that included the use of dedicated noncritical medical equipment(217, 300), assignment of dedicated cleaning personnel to the affected patient care unit(154), and increased cleaning and disinfection of frequently-touched surfaces (e.g., bedrails, charts, bedside commodes, doorknobs). A common reason given for finding environmental contamination with an MDRO was the lack of adherence to facility procedures for cleaning and disinfection. In an educational and observational intervention, which targeted a defined group of housekeeping personnel, there was a persistent decrease in the acquisition of VRE in a medical ICU(301). Therefore, monitoring for adherence to recommended environmental cleaning practices is an important determinant for success in controlling transmission of MDROs and other pathogens in the environment(274, 302).

   In the MDRO reports reviewed, enhanced environmental cleaning was frequently undertaken when there was evidence of environmental contamination and ongoing transmission. Rarely, control of the target MDRO required vacating a patient care unit for complete environmental cleaning and assessment(175, 279).

7. ***Decolonization.*** Decolonization entails treatment of persons colonized with a specific MDRO, usually MRSA, to eradicate carriage of that organism. Although some investigators have attempted to decolonize patients harboring VRE(220), few have achieved success. However, decolonization of persons carrying MRSA in their nares has proved possible with several regimens that include topical mupirocin alone or in combination with orally administered antibiotics (e.g., rifampin in combination with trimethoprim- sulfamethoxazole or ciprofloxacin) plus the use of an antimicrobial soap for bathing(303). In one report, a 3-day regimen of baths with povidone-iodine and nasal therapy with mupirocin resulted in eradication of nasal MRSA

colonization(304). These and other methods of MRSA decolonization have been thoroughly reviewed.(303, 305-307).

Decolonization regimens are not sufficiently effective to warrant routine use. Therefore, most healthcare facilities have limited the use of decolonization to MRSA outbreaks, or other high prevalence situations, especially those affecting special-care units. Several factors limit the utility of this control measure on a widespread basis: 1) identification of candidates for decolonization requires surveillance cultures; 2) candidates receiving decolonization treatment must receive follow-up cultures to ensure eradication; and 3) recolonization with the same strain, initial colonization with a mupirocin-resistant strain, and emergence of resistance to mupirocin during treatment can occur(289, 303, 308-310). HCP implicated in transmission of MRSA are candidates for decolonization and should be treated and culture negative before returning to direct patient care. In contrast, HCP who are colonized with MRSA, but are asymptomatic, and have not been linked epidemiologically to transmission, do not require decolonization.

IV. Discussion

This review demonstrates the depth of published science on the prevention and control of MDROs. Using a combination of interventions, MDROs in endemic, outbreak, and non-endemic settings have been brought under control. However, despite the volume of literature, an appropriate set of evidence-based control measures that can be universally applied in all healthcare settings has not been definitively established. This is due in part to differences in study methodology and outcome measures, including an absence of randomized, controlled trials comparing one MDRO control measure or strategy with another. Additionally, the data are largely descriptive and quasi-experimental in design(311). Few reports described preemptive efforts or prospective studies to control MDROs before they had reached high levels within a unit or facility. Furthermore, small hospitals and LTCFs are infrequently represented in the literature.
A number of questions remain and are discussed below.

Impact on other MDROS from interventions targeted to one MDRO Only one report described control efforts directed at more than one MDRO, i.e., MDR-GNB and MRSA(312). Several reports have shown either decreases or increases in other pathogens with efforts to control one MDRO. For example, two reports on VRE control efforts demonstrated an increase in MRSA following the prioritization of VRE patients to private rooms and cohort beds(161). Similarly an outbreak of *Serratia marcescens* was temporally associated with a concurrent, but unrelated, outbreak of MRSA in an NICU(313). In contrast, Wright and colleagues reported a decrease in MRSA and VRE acquisition in an ICU during and after their successful effort to eradicate an MDR-strain of *A. baumannii* from the unit(210).

Colonization with multiple MDROs appears to be common(314, 315). One study found that nearly 50% of residents in a skilled-care unit in a LTCF were colonized with a target MDRO and that 26% were co-colonized with >1 MDRO; a detailed analysis showed that risk factors for colonization varied by pathogen(316). One review of the literature(317) reported that patient risk factors associated with colonization with MRSA, VRE, MDR-GNB, *C. difficile* and *Candida sp* were the same. This review concluded that control programs that focus on only one organism or one antimicrobial drug are unlikely to succeed because vulnerable patients will continue to serve as a magnet for other MDROs.

Costs. Several authors have provided evidence for the cost-effectiveness of approaches that use ASC(153, 191, 253, 318, 319). However, the supportive evidence often relied on assumptions, projections, and estimated attributable costs of MDRO infections. Similar limitations apply to a study suggesting that gown use yields a cost benefit in controlling transmission of VRE in ICUs(320). To date, no studies have directly compared the benefits and costs associated with different MDRO control strategies.

Feasibility. The subject of feasibility, as it applies to the extrapolation of results to other healthcare settings, has not been addressed. For example, smaller hospitals and LTCFs may lack the on-site laboratory services needed to obtain ASC in a timely manner. This factor could limit the applicability of an aggressive program based on obtaining ASC and preemptive placement of patients on Contact Precautions in these settings. However, with

MDRO POLICY (CONT.)

the growing problem of antimicrobial resistance, and the recognized role of all healthcare settings for control of this problem, it is imperative that appropriate human and fiscal resources be invested to increase the feasibility of recommended control strategies in every setting.

Factors that influence selection of MDRO control measures. Although some common principles apply, the preceding literature review indicates that no single approach to the control of MDROs is appropriate for all healthcare facilities. Many factors influence the choice of interventions to be applied within an institution, including:

- *Type and significance of problem MDROs within the institution.* Many facilities have an MRSA problem while others have ESBL-producing *K. pneumoniae*. Some facilities have no VRE colonization or disease; others have high rates of VRE colonization without disease; and still others have ongoing VRE outbreaks. The magnitude of the problem also varies. Healthcare facilities may have very low numbers of cases, e.g., with a newly introduced strain, or may have prolonged, extensive outbreaks or colonization in the population. Between these extremes, facilities may have low or high levels of endemic colonization and variable levels of infection.

- *Population and healthcare-settings.* The presence of high-risk patients (e.g., transplant, hematopoietic stem-cell transplant) and special-care units (e.g. adult, pediatric, and neonatal ICUs; burn; hemodialysis) will influence surveillance needs and could limit the areas of a facility targeted for MDRO control interventions. Although it appears that MDRO transmission seldom occurs in ambulatory and outpatient settings, some patient populations (e.g., hemodialysis, cystic fibrosis) and patients receiving chemotherapeutic agents are at risk for colonization and infection with MDROs. Furthermore, the emergence of VRSA within the outpatient setting(22, 23, 25) demonstrates that even these settings need to make MDRO prevention a priority.

Differences of opinion on the optimal strategy to control MDROs. Published guidance on the control of MDROs reflects areas of ongoing debate on optimal control strategies. A key issue is the use of ASC in control efforts and preemptive use of Contact Precautions pending negative surveillance culture results(107, 321, 322). The various guidelines currently available exhibit a spectrum of approaches, which their authors deem to be evidence-based. One guideline for control of MRSA and VRE, the Society for Healthcare Epidemiology of America (SHEA) guideline from 2003(107), emphasizes routine use of ASC and Contact Precautions. That position paper does not address control of MDR-GNBs. The salient features of SHEA recommendations for MRSA and VRE control and the recommendations in this guideline for control of MDROs, including MRSA and VRE, have been compared(323); recommended interventions are similar. Other guidelines for VRE and MRSA, e.g., those proffered by the Michigan Society for Infection Control (www.msic-online.org/resource_sections/aro_guidelines), emphasize consistent practice of Standard Precautions and tailoring the use of ASC and Contact Precautions to local conditions, the specific MDROs that are prevalent and being transmitted, and the presence of risk factors for transmission. A variety of approaches have reduced MDRO rates(3, 164, 165, 209, 214, 240, 269, 324). Therefore, selection of interventions for controlling MDRO transmission should be based on assessments of the local problem, the prevalence of various MDRO and feasibility. Individual facilities should seek appropriate guidance and adopt effective measures that fit their circumstances and needs. Most studies have been in acute care settings; for non-acute care settings (e.g., LCTF, small rural hospitals), the optimal approach is not well defined.

Two-Tiered Approach for Control of MDROs. Reports describing successful control of MDRO transmission in healthcare facilities have included seven categories of interventions (Table 3). As a rule, these reports indicate that facilities confronted with an MDRO problem selected a combination of control measures, implemented them, and reassessed their impact. In some cases, new measures were added serially to further enhance control efforts. This evidence indicates that the control of MDROs is a dynamic process that requires a systematic approach tailored to the problem and healthcare setting. The nature of this evidence gave rise to the two-tiered approach to MDRO control recommended in this guideline. This approach provides the flexibility needed to prevent and control MDRO transmission in every kind of facility addressed by this guideline. Detailed recommendations for MDRO control in all healthcare settings follow and are summarized in Table 3. Table 3, which applies to all healthcare settings, contains two tiers of activities. In the first tier are the baseline level of MDRO control activities designed to ensure recognition of MDROs as a problem, involvement of healthcare administrators, and provision of safeguards for managing unidentified carriers of MDROs.

With the emergence of an MDRO problem that cannot be controlled with the basic set of infection control measures, additional control measures should be selected from the second tier of interventions presented in Table 3. Decisions to intensify MDRO control activity arise from surveillance observations and assessments of the risk to patients in various settings. Circumstances that may trigger these decisions include:

- Identification of an MDRO from even one patient in a facility or special unit with a highly vulnerable patient population (e.g., an ICU, NICU, burn unit) that had previously not encountered that MDRO.
- Failure to decrease the prevalence or incidence of a specific MDRO (e.g., incidence of resistant clinical isolates) despite infection control efforts to stop its transmission.(Statistical process control charts or other validated methods that account for normal variation can be used to track rates of targeted MDROs)(205, 325, 326).

The combination of new or increased frequency of MDRO isolates and patients at risk necessitates escalation of efforts to achieve or re-establish control, i.e., to reduce rates of transmission to the lowest possible level. Intensification of MDRO control activities should begin with an assessment of the problem and evaluation of the effectiveness of measures in current use. Once the problem is defined, appropriate additional control measures should be selected from the second tier of Table 3. A knowledgeable infection prevention and control professional or healthcare epidemiologist should make this determination. This approach requires support from the governing body and medical staff of the facility. Once interventions are implemented, ongoing surveillance should be used to determine whether selected control measures are effective and if additional measures or consultation are indicated. The result of this process should be to decrease MDRO rates to minimum levels. Healthcare facilities must not accept ongoing MDRO outbreaks or high endemic rates as the status quo. With selection of infection control measures appropriate to their situation, all facilities *can achieve* the desired goal and reduce the MDRO burden substantially.

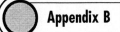

MDRO POLICY (CONT.)

V. Prevention of transmission of Multidrug Resistant Organisms (Table 3)

The CDC/HICPAC system for categorizing recommendations is as follows:

Category IA Strongly recommended for implementation and strongly supported by well-designed experimental, clinical, or epidemiologic studies.

Category IB Strongly recommended for implementation and supported by some experimental, clinical, or epidemiologic studies and a strong theoretical rationale.

Category IC Required for implementation, as mandated by federal and/or state regulation or standard.

Category II Suggested for implementation and supported by suggestive clinical or epidemiologic studies or a theoretical rationale.

No recommendation Unresolved issue. Practices for which insufficient evidence or no consensus regarding efficacy exists.

V.A.   General recommendations for all healthcare settings independent of the prevalence of multidrug resistant organism (MDRO) infections or the population served.

   V.A.1.   Administrative measures

      V.A.1.a.   Make MDRO prevention and control an organizational patient safety priority.(3, 146, 151, 154, 182, 185, 194, 205, 208, 210, 242, 327, 328) *Category IB*

      V.A.1.b.   Provide administrative support, and both fiscal and human resources, to prevent and control MDRO transmission within the healthcare organization (3, 9, 146, 152, 182-184, 208, 328, 329) *Category IB*

      V.A.1.c.   In healthcare facilities without expertise for analyzing epidemiologic data, recognizing MDRO problems, or devising effective control strategies (e.g., small or rural hospitals, rehabilitation centers, long-term care facilities [LTCFs], freestanding ambulatory centers), identify experts who can provide consultation as needed.(151, 188) *Category II*

      V.A.1.d.   Implement systems to communicate information about reportable MDROs [e.g., VRSA, VISA, MRSA, Penicillin resistant *S. pneumoniae(PRSP)*] to administrative personnel and as required by state and local health authorities (www.cdc.gov/epo/dphsi/nndsshis.htm). Refer to websites for updated requirements of local and state health departments. *Category II/IC*

V.A.1.e.   Implement a multidisciplinary process to monitor and improve healthcare personnel (HCP) adherence to recommended practices for Standard and Contact Precautions(3, 105, 182, 184, 189, 242, 273, 312, 330). *Category IB*

V.A.1.f.   Implement systems to designate patients known to be colonized or infected with a targeted MDRO and to notify receiving healthcare facilities and personnel prior to transfer of such patients within or between facilities.(87, 151) *Category IB*

V.A.1.g.   Support participation of the facility or healthcare system in local, regional, and national coalitions to combat emerging or growing MDRO problems.(41, 146, 151, 167, 188, 206, 207, 211, 331). *Category IB*

V.A.1.h.   Provide updated feedback at least annually to healthcare providers and administrators on facility and patient-care-unit trends in MDRO infections. Include information on changes in prevalence or incidence of infection, results of assessments for system failures, and action plans to improve adherence to and effectiveness of recommended infection control practices to prevent MDRO transmission.(152, 154, 159, 184, 204, 205, 242, 312, 332) *Category IB*

V.A.2.   Education and training of healthcare personnel

V.A.2.a.   Provide education and training on risks and prevention of MDRO transmission during orientation and periodic educational updates for healthcare personnel; include information on organizational experience with MDROs and prevention strategies.(38, 152, 154, 173, 176, 189, 190, 203, 204, 217, 242, 330, 333, 334) *Category IB*

V.A.3.   Judicious use of antimicrobial agents. The goal of the following recommendations is to ensure that systems are in place to promote optimal treatment of infections and appropriate antimicrobial use.

V.A.3.a.   In hospitals and LTCFs, ensure that a multidisciplinary process is in place to review antimicrobial utilization, local susceptibility patterns (antibiograms), and antimicrobial agents included in the formulary to foster appropriate antimicrobial use.(209, 212, 214, 215, 217, 242, 254, 334-339) *Category IB*

V.A.3.b. Implement systems (e.g., computerized physician order entry, comment in microbiology susceptibility report, notification from a clinical pharmacist or unit director) to prompt clinicians to use the appropriate antimicrobial agent and regimen for the given clinical situation.(156, 157, 161, 166, 174, 175, 212, 214, 218, 254, 334, 335, 337, 340-346) *Category IB*

V.A.3.b.i. Provide clinicians with antimicrobial susceptibility reports and analysis of current trends, updated at least annually, to guide antimicrobial prescribing practices.(342, 347) *Category IB*

V.A.3.b.ii. In settings that administer antimicrobial agents but have limited electronic communication system infrastructures to implement physician prompts (e.g., LTCFs, home care and infusion companies), implement a process for appropriate review of prescribed antimicrobials. Prepare and distribute reports to prescribers that summarize findings and provide suggestions for improving antimicrobial use. (342, 348, 349) *Category II*

V.A.4. Surveillance

V.A.4.a. In microbiology laboratories, use standardized laboratory methods and follow published guidance for determining antimicrobial susceptibility of targeted (e.g., MRSA, VRE, MDR-ESBLs) and emerging (e.g., VRSA, MDR-*Acinetobacter baumannii*) MDROs.(8, 154, 177, 190, 193, 209, 254, 347, 350-353) *Category IB*

V.A.4.b. In all healthcare organizations, establish systems to ensure that clinical microbiology laboratories (in-house and out-sourced) promptly notify infection control staff or a medical director/ designee when a novel resistance pattern for that facility is detected.(9, 22, 154, 162, 169) *Category IB*

V.A.4.c. In hospitals and LTCFs, develop and implement laboratory protocols for storing isolates of selected MDROs for molecular typing when needed to confirm transmission or delineate the epidemiology of the MDRO within the healthcare setting.(7, 8, 38, 140, 153, 154, 187, 190, 208, 217, 354, 355) *Category IB*

V.A.4.d.   Prepare facility-specific antimicrobial susceptibility reports as recommended by the Clinical and Laboratory Standards Institute (CLSI) (www.phppo.cdc.gov/dls/master/default.aspx); monitor these reports for evidence of changing resistance patterns that may indicate the emergence or transmission of MDROs.(347, 351, 356, 357) *Category IB/IC*

V.A.4.d.i.   In hospitals and LTCFs with special-care units (e.g., ventilator-dependent, ICU, or oncology units), develop and monitor unit-specific antimicrobial susceptibility reports.(358-361) *Category IB*

V.A.4.d.ii.   Establish a frequency for preparing summary reports based on volume of clinical isolates, with updates at least annually.(347, 362) *Category II/IC*

V.A.4.d.iii.   In healthcare organizations that outsource microbiology laboratory services (e.g., ambulatory care, home care, LTCFs, smaller acute care hospitals), specify by contract that the laboratory provide either facility-specific susceptibility data or local or regional aggregate susceptibility data in order to identify prevalent MDROs and trends in the geographic area served.(363) *Category II*

V.A.4.e.   Monitor trends in the incidence of target MDROs in the facility over time using appropriate statistical methods to determine whether MDRO rates are decreasing and whether additional interventions are needed.(152, 154, 183, 193, 205, 209, 217, 242, 300, 325, 326, 364, 365) *Category IA*

V.A.4.e.i.   Specify isolate origin (i.e., location and clinical service) in MDRO monitoring protocols in hospitals and other large multi-unit facilities with high-risk patients.(8, 38, 152-154, 217, 358, 361) *Category IB*

V.A.4.e.ii.   Establish a baseline (e.g., incidence) for targeted MDRO isolates by reviewing results of clinical cultures; if more timely or localized information is needed, perform baseline point prevalence studies of colonization in high-risk units. When possible, distinguish

MDRO POLICY (CONT.)

colonization from infection in analysis of these data.(152, 153, 183, 184, 189, 190, 193, 205, 242, 365) *Category IB*

V.A.5.   Infection control precautions to prevent transmission of MDROs

V.A.5.a.   Follow Standard Precautions during all patient encounters in all settings in which healthcare is delivered.(119, 164, 255, 315, 316) *Category IB*

V.A.5.b.   Use masks according to Standard Precautions when performing splash-generating procedures (e.g., wound irrigation, oral suctioning, intubation); when caring for patients with open tracheostomies and the potential for projectile secretions; and in circumstances where there is evidence of transmission from heavily colonized sources (e.g., burn wounds). Masks are not otherwise recommended for prevention of MDRO transmission from patients to healthcare personnel during routine care (e.g., upon room entry).(8, 22, 151, 152, 154, 189, 190, 193, 208, 240, 366) *Category IB*

V.A.5.c.   Use of Contact Precautions

V.A.5.c.i.   In *acute-care hospitals*, implement Contact Precautions routinely for all patients infected with target MDROs and for patients that have been previously identified as being colonized with target MDROs (e.g., patients transferred from other units or facilities who are known to be colonized). (11, 38, 68, 114, 151, 183, 188, 204, 217, 242, 304) *Category IB*

V.A.5.c.ii.   In LTCFs, consider the individual patient's clinical situation and prevalence or incidence of MDRO in the facility when deciding whether to implement or modify Contact Precautions in addition to Standard Precautions for a patient infected or colonized with a target MDRO. *Category II*

V.A.5.c.ii.1.   For relatively healthy residents (e.g., mainly independent) follow Standard Precautions, making sure that gloves and gowns are used for contact with uncontrolled secretions, pressure ulcers, draining wounds, stool incontinence, and ostomy tubes/bags. (78-80, 85, 151, 367, 368) *Category II*

MDRO POLICY (CONT.)

V.A.5.c.ii.2. For ill residents (e.g., those totally dependent upon healthcare personnel for healthcare and activities of daily living, ventilator-dependent) and for those residents whose infected secretions or drainage cannot be contained, use Contact Precautions in addition to Standard Precautions.(316, 369, 370) *Category II*

V.A.5.c.iii. For MDRO colonized or infected patients without draining wounds, diarrhea, or uncontrolled secretions, establish ranges of permitted ambulation, socialization, and use of common areas based on their risk to other patients and on the ability of the colonized or infected patients to observe proper hand hygiene and other recommended precautions to contain secretions and excretions.(151, 163, 371) *Category II*

V.A.5.d. In *ambulatory settings*, use Standard Precautions for patients known to be infected or colonized with target MDROs, making sure that gloves and gowns are used for contact with uncontrolled secretions, pressure ulcers, draining wounds, stool incontinence, and ostomy tubes and bags. *Category II*

V.A.5.e. In *home care settings*

- Follow Standard Precautions making sure to use gowns and gloves for contact with uncontrolled secretions, pressure ulcers, draining wounds, stool incontinence, and ostomy tubes and bags. *Category II*

- Limit the amount of reusable patient-care equipment that is brought into the home of patients infected or colonized with MDROs. When possible, leave patient-care equipment in the home until the patient is discharged from home care services. *Category II*

- If noncritical patient-care equipment (e.g., stethoscopes) cannot remain in the home, clean and disinfect items before removing them from the home, using a low to intermediate level disinfectant, or place reusable items in a plastic bag for transport

 Infection Control Program Guide

to another site for subsequent cleaning and disinfection.
Category II

V.A.5.e.i.   No recommendation is made for routine use of gloves, gowns, or both to prevent MDRO transmission in ambulatory or home care settings. *Unresolved issue*

V.A.5.e.ii.   In *hemodialysis units,* follow the "Recommendations to Prevent Transmission of Infections in Chronic Hemodialysis Patients"(372)(www.cms.hhs.gov/home/regsguidance.asp). *Category IC*

V.A.5.f.   Discontinuation of Contact Precautions. No recommendation can be made regarding when to discontinue Contact Precautions. *Unresolved issue* (See Background for discussion of options)

V.A.5.g.   Patient placement in hospitals and LTCFs

V.A.5.g.i.   When single-patient rooms are available, assign priority for these rooms to patients with known or suspected MDRO colonization or infection. Give highest priority to those patients who have conditions that may facilitate transmission, e.g., uncontained secretions or excretions.(8, 38, 110, 151, 188, 208, 240, 304) *Category IB*

V.A.5.g.ii.   When single-patient rooms are not available, cohort patients with the same MDRO in the same room or patient-care area.(8, 38, 92, 151-153, 162, 183, 184, 188, 217, 242, 304) *Category IB*

V.A.5.g.iii.   When cohorting patients with the same MDRO is not possible, place MDRO patients in rooms with patients who are at low risk for acquisition of MDROs and associated adverse outcomes from infection and are likely to have short lengths of stay. *Category II*

V.A.6.   Environmental measures

V.A.6.a.   Clean and disinfect surfaces and equipment that may be contaminated with pathogens, including those that are in close proximity to the patient (e.g., bed rails, over bed tables) and frequently-touched surfaces in the patient care environment (e.g., door knobs, surfaces in and surrounding toilets in patients' rooms) on a more frequent schedule compared to that for minimal touch surfaces (e.g., horizontal surfaces in waiting rooms).(111, 297, 373) *Category IB*

V.A.6.b. Dedicate noncritical medical items to use on individual patients known to be infected or colonized with MDROs.(38, 217, 324, 374, 375) *Category IB*

V.A.6.c. Prioritize room cleaning of patients on Contact Precautions. Focus on cleaning and disinfecting frequently touched surfaces (e.g., bedrails, bedside commodes, bathroom fixtures in the patient's room, doorknobs) and equipment in the immediate vicinity of the patient.(109, 110, 114-117, 297, 301, 373, 376, 377) *Category IB*

V.B. Intensified interventions to prevent MDRO transmission

The interventions presented below have been utilized in various combinations to reduce transmission of MDROs in healthcare facilities. Neither the effectiveness of individual components nor that of specific combinations of control measures has been assessed in controlled trials. Nevertheless, various combinations of control elements selected under the guidance of knowledgeable content experts have repeatedly reduced MDRO transmission rates in a variety of healthcare settings.

V.B.1. Indications and approach

V.B.1.a. Indications for intensified MDRO control efforts (VII.B.1.a.i and VII.B.1.a.ii) should result in selection and implementation of one or more of the interventions described in VII.B.2 to VII.B.8 below. Individualize the selection of control measures according to local considerations(8, 11, 38, 68, 114, 152-154, 183-185, 189, 190, 193, 194, 209, 217, 242, 312, 364, 365). *Category IB*

V.B.1.a.i. When incidence or prevalence of MDROs are not decreasing despite implementation of and correct adherence to the routine control measures described above, intensify MDRO control efforts by adopting one or more of the interventions described below.(92, 152, 183, 184, 193, 365) *Category IB*

V.B.1.a.ii. When the *first* case or outbreak of an epidemiologically important MDRO (e.g., VRE, MRSA, VISA, VRSA, MDR-GNB) is identified

MDRO POLICY (CONT.)

within a healthcare facility or unit.(22, 23, 25, 68, 170, 172, 184, 240, 242, 378) *Category IB*

V.B.1.b.   Continue to monitor the incidence of target MDRO infection and colonization after additional interventions are implemented. If rates do not decrease, implement more interventions as needed to reduce MDRO transmission.(11, 38, 68, 92, 152, 175, 184, 365) *Category IB*

V.B.2.   Administrative measures

V.B.2.a.   Identify persons with experience in infection control and the epidemiology of MDRO, either in house or through outside consultation, for assessment of the local MDRO problem and for the design, implementation, and evaluation of appropriate control measures (3, 68, 146, 151-154, 167, 184, 190, 193, 242, 328, 377). *Category IB*

V.B.2.b.   Provide necessary leadership, funding, and day-to-day oversight to implement interventions selected. Involve the governing body and leadership of the healthcare facility or system that have organizational responsibility for this and other infection control efforts.(8, 38, 152, 154, 184, 189, 190, 208) *Category IB*

V.B.2.c.   Evaluate healthcare system factors for their role in creating or perpetuating transmission of MDROs, including: staffing levels, education and training, availability of consumable and durable resources, communication processes, policies and procedures, and adherence to recommended infection control measures (e.g., hand hygiene and Standard or Contact Precautions). Develop, implement, and monitor action plans to correct system failures.(3, 8, 38, 152, 154, 172, 173, 175, 188, 196, 198, 199, 208, 217, 280, 324, 379, 380) *Category IB*

V.B.2.d.   During the process, update healthcare providers and administrators on the progress and effectiveness of the intensified interventions. Include information on changes in prevalence, rates of infection and colonization; results of assessments and corrective actions for system failures; degrees of adherence to recommended practices; and action plans to improve adherence to recommended infection control practices to prevent MDRO transmission.(152, 154, 159, 184, 204, 205, 312, 332, 381) *Category IB*

V.B.3.   Educational interventions

Intensify the frequency of MDRO educational programs for healthcare personnel, especially those who work in areas in which MDRO rates are not decreasing. Provide individual or unit-specific feedback when available.(3, 38, 152, 154, 159, 170, 182, 183, 189, 190, 193, 194, 204, 205, 209, 215, 218, 312) *Category IB*

V.B.4.   Judicious use of antimicrobial agents

Review the role of antimicrobial use in perpetuating the MDRO problem targeted for intensified intervention. Control and improve antimicrobial use as indicated. Antimicrobial agents that may be targeted include vancomycin, third-generation cephalosporins, and anti-anaerobic agents for VRE(217); third-generation cephalosporins for ESBLs(212, 214, 215); and quinolones and carbapenems(80, 156, 166, 174, 175, 209, 218, 242, 254, 329, 334, 335, 337, 341). *Category IB*

V.B.5.   Surveillance

V.B.5.a.   Calculate and analyze prevalence and incidence rates of targeted MDRO infection and colonization in populations at risk; when possible, distinguish colonization from infection(152, 153, 183, 184, 189, 190, 193, 205, 215, 242, 365). *Category IB*

V.B.5.a.i.   Include only one isolate per patient, not multiple isolates from the same patient, when calculating rates(347, 382). *Category II*

V.B.5.a.ii.   Increase the frequency of compiling and monitoring antimicrobial susceptibility summary reports for a targeted MDRO as indicated by an increase in incidence of infection or colonization with that MDRO. *Category II*

V.B.5.b.   Develop and implement protocols to obtain active surveillance cultures (ASC) for targeted MDROs from patients in populations at risk (e.g., patients in intensive care, burn, bone marrow/stem cell transplant, and oncology units; patients transferred from facilities known to have high

MDRO POLICY (CONT.)

MDRO prevalence rates; roommates of colonized or infected persons; and patients known to have been previously infected or colonized with an MDRO).(8, 38, 68, 114, 151-154, 167, 168, 183, 184, 187-190, 192, 193, 217, 242) *Category IB*

V.B.5.b.i.   Obtain ASC from areas of skin breakdown and draining wounds. In addition, include the following sites according to target MDROs:

V.B.5.b.i.1.   For MRSA: Sampling the anterior nares is usually sufficient; throat, endotracheal tube aspirate, percutaneous gastrostomy sites, and perirectal or perineal cultures may be added to increase the yield. Swabs from several sites may be placed in the same selective broth tube prior to transport.(117, 383, 384) *Category IB*

V.B.5.b.i.2.   For VRE: Stool, rectal, or perirectal samples should be collected.(154, 193, 217, 242)
Category IB

V.B.5.b.i.3.   For MDR-GNB: Endotracheal tube aspirates or sputum should be cultured if a respiratory tract reservoir is suspected, (e.g., *Acinetobacter* spp., *Burkholderia* spp.).(385, 386) *Category IB.*

V.B.5.b.ii.   Obtain surveillance cultures for the target MDRO from patients at the time of admission to high-risk areas, e.g., ICUs, and at periodic intervals as needed to assess MDRO transmission.(8, 151, 154, 159, 184, 208, 215, 242, 387) *Category IB*

V.B.5.c.   Conduct culture surveys to assess the efficacy of the enhanced MDRO control interventions.

V.B.5.c.i.   Conduct serial (e.g., weekly, until transmission has ceased and then decreasing frequency) unit-specific point prevalence culture surveys of the target MDRO to determine if transmission has decreased or ceased.(107, 167, 175, 184, 188, 218, 339) *Category IB*

V.B.5.c.ii.   Repeat point-prevalence culture surveys at routine intervals or at time of patient discharge or transfer until transmission has ceased.(8, 152-154, 168, 178, 190, 215, 218, 242, 388) *Category IB*

MDRO POLICY (CONT.)

V.B.5.c.iii. If indicated by assessment of the MDRO problem, collect cultures to asses the colonization status of roommates and other patients with substantial exposure to patients with known MDRO infection or colonization.(25, 68, 167, 193) *Category IB*

V.B.5.d. Obtain cultures of healthcare personnel for target MDRO when there is epidemiologic evidence implicating the healthcare staff member as a source of ongoing transmission.(153, 365) *Category IB*

V.B.6. Enhanced infection control precautions

V.B.6.a. Use of Contact Precautions

V.B.6.a.i. Implement Contact Precautions routinely for all patients colonized or infected with a target MDRO.(8, 11, 38, 68, 114, 151, 154, 183, 188, 189, 217, 242, 304) *Category IA*

V.B.6.a.ii. Because environmental surfaces and medical equipment, especially those in close proximity to the patient, may be contaminated, don gowns and gloves *before or upon entry* to the patient's room or cubicle.(38, 68, 154, 187, 189, 242) *Category IB*

V.B.6.a.iii. In LTCFs, modify Contact Precautions to allow MDRO-colonized/infected patients whose site of colonization or infection can be appropriately contained and who can observe good hand hygiene practices to enter common areas and participate in group activities.(78, 86, 151, 367) *Category IB*

V.B.6.b. When ASC are obtained as part of an intensified MDRO control program, implement Contact Precautions until the surveillance culture is reported negative for the target MDRO.(8, 30, 153, 389, 390) *Category IB*

V.B.6.c. No recommendation is made regarding universal use of gloves, gowns, or both in high-risk units in acute-care hospitals.(153, 273, 312, 320, 391) *Unresolved issue*

V.B.7. Implement policies for patient admission and placement as needed to prevent transmission of a problem MDRO.(183, 184, 189, 193, 242, 339, 392) *Category IB*

MDRO POLICY (CONT.)

V.B.7.a.i.   Place MDRO patients in single-patient rooms.(6, 151, 158, 160, 166, 170, 187, 208, 240, 282, 393-395) *Category IB*

V.B.7.a.ii.   Cohort patients with the same MDRO in designated areas (e.g., rooms, bays, patient care areas.(8, 151, 152, 159, 161, 176, 181, 183, 184, 188, 208, 217, 242, 280, 339, 344) *Category IB*

V.B.7.a.iii.   When transmission continues despite adherence to Standard and Contact Precautions and cohorting patients, assign dedicated nursing and ancillary service staff to the care of MDRO patients only. Some facilities may consider this option when intensified measures are first implemented.(184, 217, 242, 278) *Category IB*

V.B.7.a.iv.   Stop new admissions to the unit of facility if transmission continues despite the implementation of the enhanced control measures described above. (Refer to state or local regulations that may apply upon closure of hospital units or services.).(9, 38, 146, 159, 161, 168, 175, 205, 279, 280, 332, 339, 396) *Category IB*

V.B.8.   Enhanced environmental measures

V.B.8.a.   Implement patient-dedicated or single-use disposable noncritical equipment (e.g., blood pressure cuff, stethoscope) and instruments and devices.(38, 104, 151, 156, 159, 163, 181, 217, 324, 329, 367, 389, 390, 394) *Category IB*

V.B.8.b.   Intensify and reinforce training of environmental staff who work in areas targeted for intensified MDRO control and monitor adherence to environmental cleaning policies. Some facilities may choose to assign dedicated staff to targeted patient care areas to enhance consistency of proper environmental cleaning and disinfection services.(38, 154, 159, 165, 172, 173, 175, 178-181, 193, 205, 208, 217, 279, 301, 327, 339, 397) *Category IB*

V.B.8.c.   Monitor (i.e., supervise and inspect) cleaning performance to ensure consistent cleaning and disinfection of surfaces in close proximity to the patient and those likely to be touched by the patient and HCP (e.g., bedrails, carts, bedside commodes, doorknobs, faucet handles).(8, 38, 109, 111, 154, 169, 180, 208, 217, 301, 333, 398) *Category IB*

V.B.8.d. Obtain environmental cultures (e.g., surfaces, shared medical equipment) when there is epidemiologic evidence that an environmental source is associated with ongoing transmission of the targeted MDRO.(399-402) *Category IB*

V.B.8.e. Vacate units for environmental assessment and intensive cleaning when previous efforts to eliminate environmental reservoirs have failed.(175, 205, 279, 339, 403) *Category II*

V.B.9.   Decolonization

V.B.9.a. Consult with physicians with expertise in infectious diseases and/or healthcare epidemiology on a case-by-case basis regarding the appropriate use of decolonization therapy for patients or staff during limited periods of time, as a component of an intensified MRSA control program).(152, 168, 170, 172, 183, 194, 304) *Category II*

V.B.9.b. When decolonization for MRSA is used, perform susceptibility testing for the decolonizing agent against the target organism in the individual being treated or the MDRO strain that is epidemiologically implicated in transmission. Monitor susceptibility to detect emergence of resistance to the decolonizing agent. Consult with a microbiologist for appropriate testing for mupirocin resistance, since standards have not been established.(289, 290, 304, 308) *Category IB*

V.B.9.b.i.   Because mupirocin-resistant strains may emerge and because it is unusual to eradicate MRSA when multiple body sites are colonized, do not use topical mupirocin *routinely* for MRSA decolonization of patients as a component of MRSA control programs in any healthcare setting.(289, 404) *Category IB*

V.B.9.b.ii.   Limit decolonization of HCP found to be colonized with MRSA to persons who have been epidemiologically linked as a likely source of ongoing transmission to patients. Consider reassignment of HCP

MDRO POLICY (CONT.)

if decolonization is not successful and ongoing transmission to patients persists.(120, 122, 168) *Category IB*

V.B.9.c. No recommendation can be made for decolonizing patients with VRE or MDR-GNB. Regimens and efficacy of decolonization protocols for VRE and MDR-GNB have not been established.(284, 286, 288, 307, 387, 405) *Unresolved issue*

CD-ROM INSTRUCTIONS ———————————————

How to use the files on your CD-ROM

The following file names correspond with figures listed in the book, *Infection Control Program Guide.* *Note: For editorial reasons, only instructional materials have been reproduced.*

File name	Document
Definitions.pdf	Definitions
Acronyms.pdf	Acronyms
Fig1-1.rtf	Figure 1.1 Sample Infection Control Plan
Fig1-2.pdf	Figure 1.2 CDC's List of Infectious Diseases in Healthcare Settings
Fig1-4.pdf	Figure 1.4 Departmental IC Policy Matrix
Fig1-5.pdf	Figure 1.5 Sample Agenda, IC Committee
Fig2-2.rtf	Figure 2.2 IC Construction Permit
Fig2-3.rtf	Figure 2.3 Sample IC Risk Analysis
Fig2-4.rtf	Figure 2.4 IC Risk Assessment/Matrix of Precautions
Fig2-5.pdf	Figure 2.5 Administrative, Environmental, and Respiratory-protection Controls for Selected Healthcare Settings
Fig3-1.rtf	Figure 3.1 Sample IC Environmental Rounds
Fig4-1.pdf	Figure 4.1 Core Measure Indicators
Fig4-2.pdf	Figure 4.2 CDC Hand Hygiene Brochure
Fig5-3.rtf	Figure 5.3 Self-Study: MDROs
Fig6-1.rtf	Figure 6.1 Sample Avian Flu Plan
Fig6-2.rtf	Figure 6.2 Fact Sheet for Avian Flu
Fig6-3.rtf	Figure 6.3 Sample Bioterrorism Plan
Fig6-4.rtf	Figure 6.4 Sample Patient Influx
Fig7-1.rtf	Figure 7.1 CA-MRSA Fact Sheet
AppA.pdf	Appendix A – Hot list: Critical issues for Infection Control

INFECTION CONTROL PROGRAM GUIDE

Carol Shenold, RN, CIC

Create your infection control program with an expert by your side.

Written by industry insider and Joint Commission expert Carol Shenold, RN, CIC, *Infection Control Program Guide* will steer both veteran and novice infection control (IC) professionals through the challenges they face—from meeting their daily responsibilities to preparing for any Joint Commission survey. This easy-to-understand training tool provides

- an up-to-date survey of today's IC landscape

- an IC risk assessment plan

- disease-specific best-practice guidelines for ICPs and patients' families

- a bonus CD-ROM including tools to build an IC program

Stay survey-ready in the face of new threats and help educate others in the needs of IC with *Infection Control Program Guide* as your daily reference.

About HCPro

HCPro, Inc., is the premier publisher of information and training resources for the healthcare community. Our line of products includes newsletters, books, audioconferences, training handbooks, videos, online learning courses, and professional consulting seminars for specialists in health information management, compliance, finance, accreditation, quality and patient safety, nursing, pharmaceuticals, medical staff, credentialing, long-term care, physician practice, infection control, and safety.

Visit the Healthcare Marketplace at *www.hcmarketplace.com* for information on any of our products or to sign up for one of our free online e-zines.

HCPro is not affiliated in any way with The Joint Commission, which owns the JCAHO and Joint Commission trademarks.

ICPG

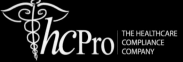

THE HEALTHCARE COMPLIANCE COMPANY

200 Hoods Lane | Marblehead, MA 01945
www.hcmarketplace.com

ISBN 978-1-57839-958-1

9 781578 399581